# The Menopause
What you need to know

# THE MENOPAUSE
## WHAT YOU NEED TO KNOW

Dr Margaret Rees
Professor David W. Purdie
Dr Sally Hope

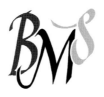

Published by BMS Publications Ltd
on behalf of
THE BRITISH MENOPAUSE SOCIETY,
4-6 Eton Place, Marlow, Bucks SL7 2QA, UK

First published 2003

© BMS Publications Ltd 2003

ISBN 0-9536228-2-7

Published by BMS Publications Ltd on behalf of
The British Menopause Society
4-6 Eton Place, Marlow
Bucks SL7 2QA, UK

The British Menopause Society is a
Registered Charity, No. 101544

# CONTENTS

# ABOUT THIS BOOK

Women and their doctors are divided over how to approach the menopause. Some feel it is a natural event, which should not normally need medical treatment. Others believe that the many long term effects on a woman's bone, heart, blood vessels and nerves which occur after the ovaries stop producing hormones represent an important, and often under-treated, medical condition.

However, whatever our beliefs, there is no doubt that many women experience considerable stress around the time that their monthly periods end. There is also growing evidence that the change in hormone production can lead to conditions such as thinning bones, clogged arteries and memory loss. These have a major effect on the quality of many women's lives.

One problem in understanding the menopause is that it is a relatively new experience. Until the 19th century, most women simply did not live long enough to reach the menopause, and doctors only started studying it about 60 years ago.

Medical research aims to understand the mechanisms of the changes that occur when a woman's periods stop. In particular, we need to know more about the negative effects of the menopause and to develop safe, effective and affordable ways of reducing or preventing them.

The aim of this book is to provide unbiased and non-promotional information about managing the menopause, but the ultimate decision about what course to take should only be made after talking to a health professional.

*The Menopause: What you need to know* is based on the British Menopause Society Handbook for doctors. Menopause specialists wrote the Handbook for family doctors, gynaecologists, nurses and other health professionals. The first edition was produced in 1994 and it was last updated in 2002. Its success prompted the British Menopause Society to produce a version for those who actually have to face the menopause and its consequences.

Where possible we have avoided using medical language, but we have tried to include definitions of words that a health professional might use. There is a Word List at the end of the book giving definitions of these terms. In the sections at the end of each chapter entitled "Sources of information" you will find a series of book, journal and web site references. These are not exhaustive lists but aim to show what is available. The journals are listed on Medline and can be accessed using the following web site: http://www.ncbi.nlm.nih.gov/entrez/query.fcgi.

The British Menopause Society (a registered charity) was founded in 1989 as an independent scientific society for health professionals. Its aims are to raise awareness about the menopause and improve the treatment that menopausal women receive. It organises clinical and scientific meetings and produces a scientific journal for healthcare professionals.

*Dr Margaret Rees*
*Professor David W. Purdie*
*Dr Sally Hope*
*January 2003*

*Acknowledgements*

We thank the Council members of the British Menopause Society and other medical experts who contributed to the doctors' Handbook and to this version. We also thank the following non-medical people who reviewed the book and gave us helpful comments: Ray Anson, Oxford; Lesley Cornes, Ringmer; Pauline Crook, Ringmer; Katherine Evans, Flitwick; Sheila George, High Wycombe; Christine Gillson, Oxford; Robert Gillson, Oxford; Wendy Hirsh, Ringmer; Carol Leonard, Oxford; Dee Nudds, Oxford; Susan Pearce, Lewes.

Liz Wager of Sideview reworked the text for this version and Simon Brown produced the book on behalf of the British Menopause Society.

# CHAPTER 1
# WHAT IS THE MENOPAUSE?

The menopause is the time when a woman's monthly periods finally stop. The average age of the menopause is 51. The word menopause comes from the Greek words *menos*, meaning a month, and *pausos* an ending. Because it is not always possible to define the point at which periods stop, doctors have agreed the following definitions:

**Menopause**
Because menopause means the final monthly period, it can only be recognised after the event. In medical terms, the menopause is considered to have occurred after a woman has gone for 12 months without having periods, so long as there is no other reason for this. If a woman is still having periods, even if irregular, the menopause has not yet occurred.

**Premenopause**
This term can be used to mean either just one or two years before the menopause, or the whole of a woman's reproductive life before the menopause. In this book, we use it to mean the entire phase from a woman's first to her last monthly period.

**Perimenopause**
This term describes the time from when a woman first notices menopausal symptoms, such as hot flushes or irregular periods, until 12 months after her last monthly period.

**Postmenopause**
This means the time after a woman's last menstrual period. For

11

women whose menopause is caused by oophorectomy (operation to remove the ovaries) or chemotherapy the start of the postmenopause may be obvious. For those who have a natural menopause it cannot be determined until they have gone for 12 months without periods.

### Menopause transition
This is the time just before the final menstrual period. Many women have irregular periods during this phase. The length of the menopause transition varies from woman to woman and may last several years.

### Climacteric
This term refers to a woman's transition from the reproductive to the non-reproductive state. Strictly speaking, the menopause is just one event that occurs during the climacteric, just as menarche (when monthly periods start) is just one event within puberty.

### Climacteric syndrome
Many, but by no means all, women experience symptoms around the menopause. The collection of symptoms is sometimes referred to as the climacteric syndrome.

### Premature or early menopause
The average age when most women's periods stop is around 51. This is considered a normal menopause, but there is considerable variation either side of this age, and between women in different countries. Furthermore, estimates of age of menopause in developing countries may not always be accurate. It is therefore quite difficult to define a premature menopause. In developed countries such as Britain menopause occurring before a woman is 45 is considered premature.

### Induced menopause
This term is used to describe a menopause caused by surgery (such as an oophorectomy), chemotherapy, radiotherapy or other medical treatment. It contrasts with the natural or spontaneous menopause, which would otherwise have occurred when a woman reached the age of about 51.

## What causes the menopause?

A woman's monthly menstrual periods stop when her ovaries (the female reproductive organs) stop working or are removed. The timing of a woman's menopause may be set even before she is born, since slow growth as a baby during the last part of pregnancy seems to be linked to an early menopause. Genetic factors are important, since women with Down's syndrome tend to have an earlier menopause, and Japanese women tend to have a later one. Environmental factors may also play a part. Women who smoke tend to have their menopause up to three years earlier on average than non-smokers.

### Role of the ovaries

The ovaries are controlled by two hormones produced by the pituitary, which is a small gland just underneath the brain. These hormones are called FSH (follicle stimulating hormone) and LH (luteinising hormone). FSH and LH are controlled by another hormone called GnRH (gonadotrophin releasing hormone), which is produced in the brain itself. GnRH in turn is affected by chemicals produced by the ovaries. The ovaries produce the two female hormones oestradiol and progesterone. In premenopausal women, the levels of these sex hormones in the blood change regularly over the course of the monthly menstrual cycle and also regulate the levels of GnRH. The interaction between the brain, the pituitary gland and the ovaries is explained in Figure 1.1 on the following page. The anatomy of the female pelvic organs is shown in Figure 1.2.

When the ovaries are functioning they also secrete a small protein called inhibin, high levels of which stop the secretion of GnRH. When a woman is fertile, her ovaries normally release one egg cell at every cycle – this is known as ovulation. This usually happens around day 14 of a 28-day cycle. Changes in hormone levels during the cycle are illustrated in Figure 1.3 on page 16.

The egg cells (or oocytes) are laid down in a woman's ovaries before she is born. From that point on, the number decreases until, about 50 years later, very few are left. As a woman ages her ovaries gradually become less responsive to FSH and LH and produce less oestrogen. Although she may still have monthly bleeds, the number of anovulatory menstrual cycles, when no egg is released,

13

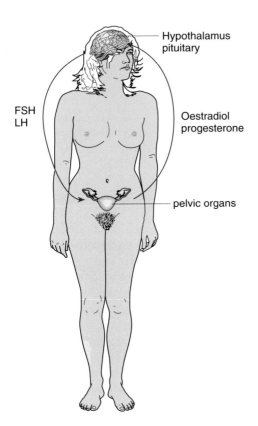

Hypothalamus
pituitary

FSH
LH

Oestradiol
progesterone

pelvic organs

Figure 1.1.
Interactions between the
hypothalamus, pituitary
and ovaries.

gradually increases towards the menopause.

Around the menopause the levels of female sex hormones may fluctuate almost daily, but over time there is a gradual increase in levels of FSH, then of LH in the blood, and a fall in oestradiol and inhibin levels. Consistently low levels of oestrogen cause a woman's periods to stop. FSH levels above 30 international units per litre of blood are usually a sign that the ovaries are failing and that the menopause is nearing or has occurred. In premenopausal women FSH levels are usually 10 international units per litre of blood or less.

Figure 1.4 on page 17 illustrates the fluctuation in FSH levels around the menopause.

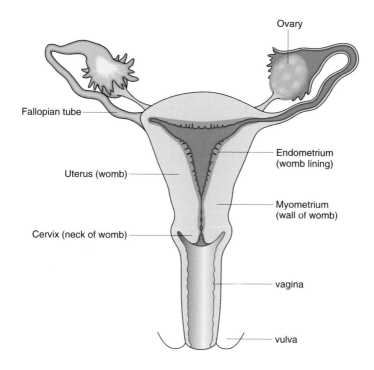

Figure 1.2 . Anatomy of the female pelvic organs.

### Early (premature) menopause
If the ovaries fail before age 45, the condition is called a premature menopause. If it is because of natural causes, it is called primary premature ovarian failure. If the ovaries stop working because of treatment, such as radiotherapy or chemotherapy, it is called secondary premature ovarian failure. In most cases the causes of an early menopause are unknown.

**Primary premature ovarian failure** can be caused by:
● Abnormal chromosomes (eg, Down's syndrome and Turner's syndrome).
● Autoimmune diseases (which can be associated with diabetes and under-active thyroid).
● Abnormal hormone production or hormone receptors.

15

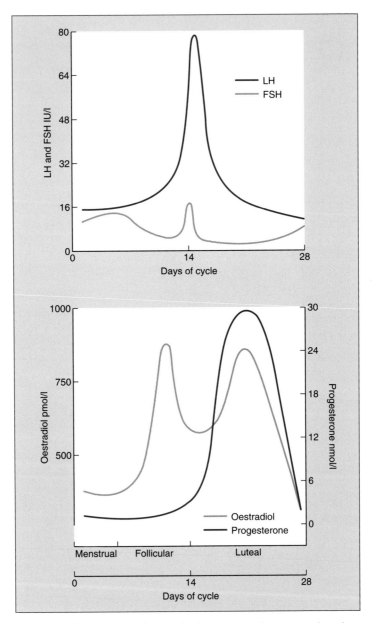

Figure 1.3. Hormone levels during a normal menstrual cycle.

- Metabolic or biochemical disorders (eg, galactosemia, a very rare disorder of sugar metabolism).

**Secondary premature ovarian failure** can be caused by:
Radiotherapy or chemotherapy for cancer (the effects depend on the dose given and the woman's age).
- Surgical removal of both ovaries (sometimes called bilateral oophorectomy).
- Surgical removal of the womb (hysterectomy). Sometimes the ovaries fail immediately after hysterectomy, in other cases they continue to work for a while, but some women will experience an early menopause. Diagnosing the menopause after a hysterectomy is difficult, since the woman will no longer be having periods and she may not have typical menopausal symptoms such as hot flushes.
- Infection (eg, tuberculosis or mumps). This is extremely rare and most cases of mumps only cause a temporary loss of ovary function if any.

Women who have an early menopause and who do not receive oestrogen replacement have a higher risk of osteoporosis (or brittle bone disease) and heart disease but are less likely to have breast cancer. Women who have an early menopause should normally be offered HRT (hormone replacement therapy) until the average age

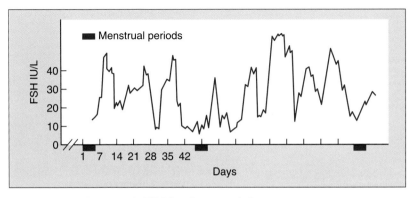

Figure 1.4. FSH levels around the menopause.

17

of menopause (51), unless there are reasons why they cannot take it. This does not increase the risk of breast cancer any more than for women who are still having their periods (see chapter 6).

**Why does the menopause happen?**
Women lose their fertility much earlier than other animal species and some scientists believe that the human menopause evolved to protect women and their children from the dangers of late childbearing.

One important difference between us and other mammals is that human children depend on their parents for a longer period of their lives. Our highly evolved brain means that, at birth, human babies have larger heads than other species, which makes childbirth more difficult. Because of this, human babies spend a relatively short time in the womb and are therefore born at a less developed stage than other mammals.

The risks of childbirth to both the mother and baby increase as the mother gets older. For the older woman there may therefore be little survival advantage in further pregnancies, when her earlier children still depend on her for their survival.

Another explanation is that humans have evolved into extended family groups, and the presence of postmenopausal grandmothers might help their daughters to raise their grandchildren.

However, not all scientists accept these evolutionary explanations. Others believe that the menopause is simply because of the fact that humans live much longer than other mammals of a similar size. All mammals form their female reproductive cells before birth, so we start life with a limited number of eggs, and our ovaries may simply run out of eggs as our bodies age.

**The ageing population**
Women born in the UK can expect to live, on average, for 81 years. Thus, most British women can expect more than 30 years of life after the menopause. Because more and more people will live until the age of 100, the menopause can even be considered to be a mid-life stage.

The increase in life expectancy combined with falling birth rates means that the proportion of older people in the population is growing, as indicated in Figure 1.5. By 2015 the over-60s will

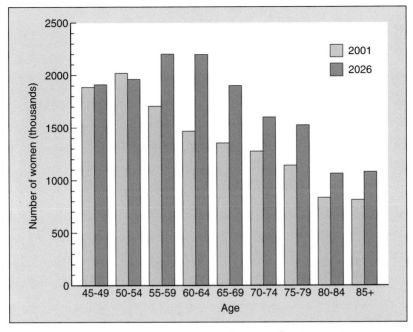

Figure 1.5. The increase in the number of women aged over 45 predicted to occur in the UK by the year 2026. The columns on the left show figures for 2001; those on the right show the numbers for 2026. (Adapted from Office for National Statistics and Government Actuaries Department 2002.)

outnumber the under-20s for the first time in our history.

By 2025:

● Worldwide life expectancy will have risen to 73 years - a 50% improvement on the 1955 global average of only 48 years.

● The number of people aged over 65 will have risen from 420 million in 2000 to 825 million, ie, from 7% to 10% of the total population.

● There will never have been so many people aged over 80, and women will form the majority.

## Sources of information

### Journal articles
Burger HG. The endocrinology of the menopause. J Steroid Biochem Mol Biol 1999; 69: 31-35.

Cooper GS, Thorp JM Jr. FSH levels in relation to hysterectomy and to unilateral oophorectomy. Obstet Gynecol 1999; 94: 969-972.

Ebbiary NA, Lenton EA, Cooke ID. Hypothalamic-pituitary ageing: progressive increase in FSH and LH concentrations throughout the reproductive life in regularly menstruating women. Clin Endocrinol 1994; 41: 199-206.

Gold EB, Bromberger J, Crawford S, et al. Factors associated with age at natural menopause in a multiethnic sample of midlife women. Am J Epidemiol 2001; 153: 865-874.

Hardy R, Kuh D. Does early growth influence timing of the menopause? Evidence from a British birth cohort. Hum Reprod 2002; 17: 2474-2479.

Kalantaridou SN, Nelson LM. Premature ovarian failure is not premature menopause. Ann N Y Acad Sci 2000; 900: 393-402.

Robertson DM, Burger HG. Reproductive hormones: ageing and the perimenopause. Acta Obstet Gynecol Scand 2002; 81: 612-616.

Utian WH. The international menopause society menopause-related terminology definitions. Climacteric 1999; 2: 284-286.

### Web sites
Office for National Statistics and Government Actuaries Department, UK. http://www.gad.gov.uk

US Census Bureau. World population information. http://www.census.gov/ipc/www/world.html

World Health Report 1998. WHO. http://www.who.int/whr/1998/exsum98e.htm

# CHAPTER 2
# SYMPTOMS OF THE MENOPAUSE

Changes in hormone levels, particularly a fall in oestrogen, can cause symptoms around the menopause. About 70% of women experience symptoms such as hot flushes and night sweats. Some women also report psychological symptoms; these may be linked to their other symptoms, or may be a reaction to menstrual changes or other life events. Such symptoms include tiredness, lack of energy, depressed mood, aches and pains, and reduced interest in sex.

There are probably cultural differences in women's attitudes to the menopause. For example, Japanese women report fewer symptoms than Americans. Furthermore, a recent Swedish study showed that women with a higher education and who exercised regularly were more likely to be symptom-free.

## Vasomotor symptoms

Hot flushes and night sweats - known as vasomotor symptoms - are the most common symptoms of the menopause and can occur before the last period. Hot flushes occur most often in the first year after the final period.

They are caused by a malfunction in the body's normal methods of controlling its temperature. Women with hot flushes are unable to control body heat normally (the so-called "vasomotor" response).

Hot flushes can occur at any time of the day or night. Night-time flushes and sweats can disturb the woman's sleep patterns which may lead to insomnia, irritability and difficulties with memory and concentration.

## Sexual problems

Changes in sexual behaviour and activity are not uncommon in menopausal women. Both men and women gradually lose interest in sex as they get older, but the decrease seems to be more marked in women. Older women may experience less desire for sex, find it harder to become sexually aroused and to have an orgasm, and sex may be painful for them.

These changes are caused by several different factors. Lower oestrogen levels cause vaginal dryness, which may make sex uncomfortable. Hormone levels may also affect a woman's sensory perception. Interest in sex may also decrease if a woman's sleep is disturbed by night sweats and hot flushes, or if she feels depressed. Menopausal symptoms may also contribute to difficulties in relationships, which makes matters worse. But the problems may not always lie with the woman, and male sexual problems, such as loss of libido and erection problems, should not be overlooked.

## Psychological symptoms

Psychological symptoms, including depressed mood, anxiety, irritability, mood swings, tiredness and lack of energy, have been linked to the menopause. However, large population surveys suggest that most women do not have major mood changes around their menopause and there is no clear evidence that changes in hormone levels can cause depression.

However, around the same time as her menopause, women may experience stressful events such as:

- Parents ageing and becoming less independent
- Death of parents, relatives or friends
- Loss of a partner through death, separation or divorce
- Lack of social support
- Children leaving home or "empty nest syndrome"
- Worries over children's education, jobs or relationships
- Poor health
- Demanding workload or job insecurity
- Money problems
- Coming to terms with ageing in a culture that values youth and fertility

These factors, together with the physical changes of the

22

menopause, can combine to make a woman feel stressed and unable to cope. Because the factors are different for every woman, you have to make your own choice and be comfortable with it. Treatments might include counselling, dietary and exercise advice, psychological therapy, HRT, antidepressants, or a combination of these.

## Sources of information

### Journal articles
Berman JR, Goldstein I. Female sexual dysfunction. Urol Clin North Am 2001; 28: 405-416.

Bromberger JT, Meyer PM, Kravitz HM, et al . Psychologic distress and natural menopause: a multiethnic community study. Am J Public Health 2001; 91: 1435-1442.

Dennerstein L, Lehert P, Dudley E, Guthrie J. Factors contributing to positive mood during the menopausal transition. J Nerv Ment Dis 2001; 189: 84-89.

Laumann EO, Paik A, Rosen RC. Sexual dysfunction in the United States: prevalence and predictors. JAMA 1998; 281: 537-544.

Lock M, Kaufert P. Menopause, local biologies, and cultures of aging. Am J Human Biol 2001; 13: 494-504.

Stadberg E, Mattsson LA, Milsom I. Factors associated with climacteric symptoms and the use of hormone replacement therapy. Acta Obstet Gynecol Scand  2000; 79: 286-292.

Stearns V, Ullmer L, Loçpez JF, et al. Hot flushes. Lancet 2002; 360: 1851-1861.

## CHAPTER 3
# LONG-TERM EFFECTS OF THE MENOPAUSE

The long-term effects of the menopause probably affect the quality, and even the length, of women's lives more than the short-term symptoms. This is why you need to take care of your own health. The overall effects on women's health also pose an economic burden on the health system. However, these effects may be hard to measure, since they often remain clinically silent for many years.

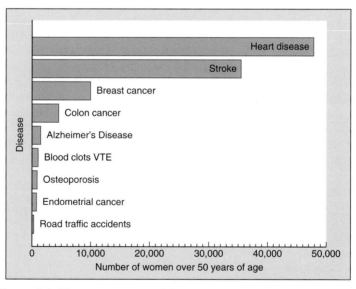

Figure 3.1. The main causes of death in women over the age of 50 in England and Wales in 2000. The numbers for osteoporosis and Alzheimer's disease are probably underestimates because these are often not accurately reported on death certificates. As in other Western societies, heart disease and stroke are the major killers.

## Cardiovascular disease

Cardiovascular disease means any disease of the heart or blood vessels. The major diseases in this group are heart attacks and strokes. Although cardiovascular disease rarely kills women under 60 it is the most common cause of death in older women. Heart disease and stroke together account for about one third of deaths.

There is some evidence that women are more likely to suffer from blocked arteries after the menopause. Studies of women who have had an operation to remove their ovaries (oophorectomy) suggest that they are 2-3 times more likely to have a coronary (heart attack) than women of the same age who still have their ovaries and are premenopausal.

### Coronary heart disease

Coronary heart disease (CHD) is the biggest single cause of death in British women. Although it accounts for about one in five of all female deaths, it is still often considered, wrongly, to be largely a male problem. The rate of CHD increases after the menopause but the rate of increase is remarkably similar in both men and women over 50. Heart attacks are more common in men, because their increase in rate with age starts earlier than for women. While some studies have suggested that women have more problems than men after a heart attack, others have shown that men are far more likely to suffer another fatal attack.

A heart attack (or myocardial infarction) happens when one or more of the major (coronary) arteries supplying the heart muscle with blood become blocked. This starves the heart muscle of oxygen so that it cannot pump properly. Arteries usually become blocked because a blood clot (or thrombus) forms in a vessel that has been narrowed by a build-up of fatty material called a plaque (see Figure 3.2). Doctors used to believe that cholesterol was a major cause of narrowing arteries (or atherosclerosis). Scientists now recognise that the process is more complex and may also involve damage to the artery through other processes such as high blood pressure and inflammation of the blood vessel lining.

Drugs called statins can help to reduce cholesterol levels in the blood and may also protect the artery walls. It is not clear whether some types of HRT may prevent heart disease or not (see Chapter 6 for more details about this).

25

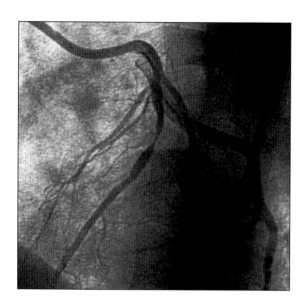

Figure 3.2. Angiogram or x-ray showing a blocked coronary artery. The artery flowing from top middle to lower left has narrowed to a point where blood flow is almost impossible.

Stopping smoking, keeping body weight normal, following a healthy diet (low in cholesterol and high in fresh fruit and vegetables) and taking regular exercise can help reduce the risk of heart disease in women of all ages.

**Stroke**
Strokes kill large numbers of women and leave many others with serious disabilities. A stroke happens when part of the brain is starved of oxygen. The most common cause of stroke is when an artery supplying the brain gets blocked by a blood clot. Strokes can also be caused by bleeding (haemorrhage) in the brain. Because both heart attacks and strokes can be caused by narrowed arteries and blood clots, some of the risk factors are similar for both. However, high blood pressure (hypertension) is particularly linked with strokes and high cholesterol levels (hyperlipidaemia) may be slightly less important.

**Effects of the menopause on the risk of cardiovascular disease**
Changes in lipids, artery lining (or endothelium), blood clotting, and response to insulin have all been described at the menopause.

These can affect the risk of developing cardiovascular disease. Details are given below.

**Lipids.** Blood contains some fatty substances or lipids. Most people have heard of cholesterol and believe it causes narrowing of the arteries. However, we now know that there are several forms of cholesterol, such as low- and high-density lipoprotein (LDL and HDL) which can have different effects. While high levels of LDL in the blood increase the risk of blocked arteries and heart disease, HDL actually protects against these.

Postmenopausal women who do not use HRT generally have higher levels of LDL (bad cholesterol) and triglycerides (another type of blood fat) than premenopausal women. They also have lower levels of HDL (good cholesterol). In the worst cases, this change in blood lipid levels can increase the risk of heart disease by about 20%.

**Blood clotting (coagulation).** A healthy system is one in which blood clots only if we are injured. The process of forming a blood clot involves many different chemicals, which normally circulate in an inactive form in the blood. Clots that form inside the body can cause heart attacks and strokes. Some of the risk of cardiovascular disease can be predicted by measuring the levels of certain substances involved in clotting such as fibrinogen, plasminogen activator inhibitor (PAI-1) and Factor VII. After the menopause the levels of all these chemicals in the blood usually rise.

**Insulin sensitivity.** Insulin is produced by the pancreas. It is involved with the release and storage of energy from carbo-hydrates (sugars) in the form of glucose. People with diabetes do not produce enough insulin, or they become resistant to its effects. After the menopause, women's resistance to the effects of insulin gradually increases. However, most studies have found little or no immediate effect of the menopause itself on insulin production or the way in which the body uses glucose.

**Endothelial function.** The endothelium is the name of the inner lining of blood vessels. This part of the artery is important because it controls the size of the vessel which will then affect blood flow.

An increase in the size, or diameter, of a blood vessel is called vasodilatation, a decrease is called vasoconstriction. These terms refer to active changes caused by muscles in the vessel wall, rather than the irreversible accumulation of fatty deposits or plaque. Postmenopausal women with normal cholesterol and glucose levels have less vasodilatation than premenopausal women.

**Inflammatory markers.** The body produces certain chemicals in response to injury. These help protect against infection and to heal wounds. However, they may also cause unwanted blood clots which may cause heart attacks and strokes. Levels can change after the menopause and may increase the risk of cardiovascular disease.

**Body weight.** Obesity increases the risk of cardiovascular disease. Most women gain weight around the menopause, and may therefore increase their risk of a heart attack, stroke or diabetes. An increase in weight can also put up blood pressure, but there is no sign that the menopause itself causes raised blood pressure.

## Osteoporosis (brittle bones)

As men and women get old their bones become lighter and more brittle; this can lead to osteoporosis (see Figure 3.3). Although all elderly people experience bone loss, the change occurs much faster in women after the menopause. This explains why one in three women suffers from osteoporosis - and only one in 12 men.

Osteoporosis increases the risk of breaking the bones in the wrist, hip or spine. Such fractures can have a major effect on a person's quality of life and independence, and may even shorten their life. Treating such fractures, and caring for people with osteoporosis, also accounts for considerable costs to the health service and to society. By the age of 80 most women will have had at least one fracture. Every day the National Health Service in the UK spends £5 million (7.5 million Euros) on caring for people with osteoporotic fractures.

Worldwide, the number of hip fractures resulting from osteoporosis is expected to treble by the middle of the next century, from 1.7 million in 1990 to 6.3 million by 2050 because of increasing life expectancy (see chapter 1). Population changes over the next 50 years will lead to increases in the number of elderly women.

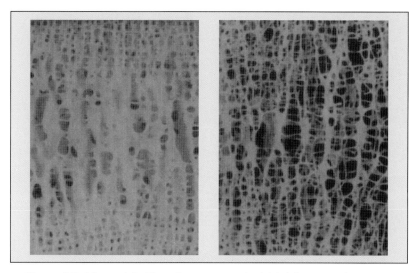

Figure 3.3. Normal (left) and osteoporotic (right) bone in the spine.
Osteoporotic bone is less dense and strong than normal bone.

## The pattern of bone loss

Bone density increases during the teens and reaches a peak
sometime in the twenties. This peak bone density is sustained for
some years but starts to decline during the mid-forties. For 6-10
years after the menopause women lose bone rapidly. After that,
bone loss continues but at a much slower rate. Once bone reaches
a certain stage, even a minor injury will cause it to break. This
pattern of bone loss in women and men is illustrated in Figure 3.4
on the following page.

Three factors determine whether a woman develops
osteoporosis. These are:
● how strong her bones were when she was in her 20s (her peak
bone mass)
● how fast her bones thin after the menopause
● and how long she lives after the menopause

Men generally develop osteoporosis much later than women
because they have a much higher peak bone mass and do not
suffer the rapid loss that occurs after the menopause. Men do not
have the equivalent of the female menopause with a sudden fall in

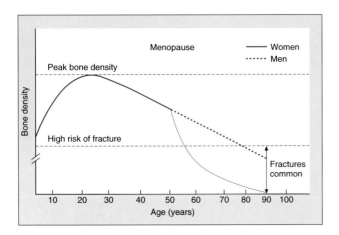

Figure 3.4. The pattern of bone loss in women and men.

hormone levels; testosterone gradually declines with age.

Factors that probably increase peak bone mass are:

- a diet high in calcium and vitamin D
- not smoking (especially in your teens)
- taking weight-bearing exercise (eg, jogging)

However there have been no trials in teenagers to confirm that these really do prevent osteoporosis in later life.

### Risk factors for osteoporosis

Risk of osteoporosis varies among ethnic groups and white people suffer more fractures than Afro-Caribbeans. Osteoporosis is probably not caused by a single gene, but a woman's risk of developing it may be due to variations in several genes. Bone density is largely (about 80%) determined by inherited factors, with lifestyle factors playing a lesser role.

Certain groups of women have a high risk of suffering a fracture because of osteoporosis (see Table 3.1). However, it is not always easy to assess the risk for an individual woman, because the effects of some risk factors are small. The most important factors seem to be an early menopause before the age of 45 (see chapter 1), long-term corticosteroid use (particularly tablets such as prednisolone but possibly the use of steroids in asthma inhalers as well), long-term immobility, previous fractures and osteoporosis occurring in a mother or a sister.

30

| | |
|---|---|
| **Genetic** | Family history (especially mother or sister) |
| **Constitutional** | Low body weight<br>Early menopause (under 45) |
| **Environmental** | Cigarette smoking<br>Alcohol abuse<br>Low calcium intake<br>Sedentary life style (not enough exercise) |
| **Drugs** | Corticosteroids (more than 5 mg<br>    prednisolone or equivalent daily) |
| **Diseases** | Anorexia nervosa<br>Rheumatoid arthritis<br>Neuromuscular disease<br>Chronic liver disease<br>Malabsorption syndromes<br>Hyperparathyroidism (overactive parathyroid)<br>Hyperthyroidism (overactive thyroid) |

Table 3.1. Risk factors for osteoporosis.

The effect of the injected contraceptive Depo-Provera (DMPA) on bone density is controversial. The best evidence suggests that DMPA causes a 5-10% loss of bone, but this is not progressive. DMPA is probably safe for women of normal build, with a good diet and exercise, but may pose a risk for those with a family history of osteoporosis and a personal history of poor diet, little exercise and smoking. In such cases, a bone density scan may be arranged. If this shows a woman to be at risk of osteoporosis, an alternative method of contraception may be considered. DMPA should probably be stopped at age 40 to allow the menstrual cycle to resume for the last 10 years or so to the menopause. The effects of DMPA on teenagers who have not yet reached their peak bone mass is currently being studied. It is undoubtedly a very effective form of contraception.

**Effects of osteoporosis**

The main consequence of osteoporosis is broken bones. The most common bones to break are those in the arm/wrist, hip and spine. Falling on an outstretched hand often causes Colles fractures of the radius bone in the wrist, which are painful and severely limit the use of the arm and hand.

Hip fractures in young women are unusual and most commonly caused by road accidents. However, in older women with brittle bones they can be caused by falls or even spontaneously. Women are twice as likely to fracture a hip as men. A British woman at menopause has a one in eight (12%) risk of breaking her hip during her life. Broken hips cause more deaths, disability and medical costs than all other osteoporotic fractures combined. A woman who has broken her hip is 20% more likely to die the following year than if she had not broken it. One in two patients with a broken hip will have some permanent disability or loss of independence.

The effects of osteoporosis on the spine (vertebral fractures) are hard to measure because there are often no symptoms until the spine has become seriously deformed. Vertebral fractures often cause non-specific back pain and up to 90% are never seen by doctors. Multiple fractures cause height loss and a characteristic stooping (the so-called "dowager's hump"). They can cause considerable pain and loss of quality of life and may eventually restrict breathing. Presence of one vertebral fracture suggests a high risk of future fractures both in the spine and elsewhere. The main goal of osteoporosis research is to prevent the first fracture.

## Changes in the vagina and urinary system

Women's urinary and reproductive systems are both affected by oestrogen levels. Following the decrease in oestrogen after the menopause, a number of changes take place:

- The vagina shortens and becomes less elastic
- The inner surface of the vagina gets flatter
- Blood supply to the vaginal lining (epithelium) decreases, so it becomes thinner
- Vaginal secretions decrease
- The risk of vaginal and bladder infections increases
- The tube that carries urine out of the bladder (urethra) starts to work less well

**Vaginal**
- Dryness
- Burning
- Itching (pruritis)
- Pain/discomfort during sex
- Prolapse or a feeling of something coming down (when internal organs such as the womb, bladder and bowel sink into the vagina)

**Urinary**
- Urgency, or uncontrollable wish to pass water
- Passing water more frequently
- Pain on passing water
- Water infection
- Incontinence or leaking
- Difficulty in passing water

Table 3.2. Urogenital changes and symptoms.

A summary of changes and symptoms affecting the vagina and urinary system is shown in Table 3.2.

## Changes to connective tissue
Collagen is an important protein in skin, hair, nails and tendons. Oestrogen levels affect its production. After the menopause, the body produces less collagen. This causes the skin to become dryer, thinner, wrinkled and less elastic. Women may also notice that their skin breaks and bruises more easily after the menopause. These changes are thought to be largely due to the decline in collagen levels. Some studies have shown that the inner and outer skin layers (dermis and epidermis) are thicker and contain more collagen in postmenopausal women taking HRT than in those that do not. However, another study found that the rate of collagen production did not seem to be linked to HRT use.

## Sources of information

### Journal articles

Burns A, Byrne EJ, Maurer K. Alzheimer's disease. Lancet 2002; 360: 163-165.

Gorodeski GI. Update on cardiovascular disease in post-menopausal women. Best Pract Res Clin Obstet Gynaecol 2002;16: 329-55.

van Staa TP, Dennison EM, Leufkens HG, Cooper C. Epidemiology of fractures in England and Wales. Bone 2001; 29: 517-522.

Versi E, Harvey MA, Cardozo L, et al. Urogenital prolapse and atrophy at menopause: a prevalence study. Int Urogynecol J Pelvic Floor Dysfunct 2001; 12: 107-110.

### Web sites

Department of Health. National Service Framework for Older People 2001. Department of Health, PO Box 410, Wetherby LS23 7LN. http://www.doh.gov.uk/nsf/olderpeople.htm

Department of Health . Quick reference primary care guide on the prevention and treatment of osteoporosis 1998. Department of Health, PO Box 410, Wetherby LS23 7LN.   http://www.open.gov.uk/doh/osteop.htm

Office for National Statistics. Mortality statistics cause review of the Registrar General on deaths by cause, sex and age, in England and Wales, 2000 : Series DH2 no 27. http://www.statistics.gov.uk

Royal College of Physicians. Osteoporosis: clinical guidelines for prevention and treatment. London, Royal College of Physicians 1999. http://www.rcplondon.ac.uk/files/osteosummary.pdf

Royal College of Physicians. Osteoporosis: clinical guidelines for prevention and treatment. Update on pharmacological interventions and an alogorithm for management. London, Royal College of Physicians 2000. http://www.rcplondon.ac.uk/pubs/wp_osteo_update.htm

# CHAPTER 4
# UNDERSTANDING YOUR DOCTOR'S TESTS

Your doctor might suggest that you have some tests to check
- hormone levels
- the womb if you have unexpected vaginal bleeding
- your bones

You should discuss any tests with your doctor, and ask for the results to be explained to you. A summary of the different tests which might be used appears on the next page in Table 4.1.

## Hormone tests
Sometimes, problems occurring around the menopause have nothing to do with oestrogen levels, so it is important to rule out other conditions. Your doctor might order blood or urine tests if she/he suspects this might be the case, or if you have menopausal symptoms that are not responding to HRT (see Table 4.1).

## Examining the womb and its lining
Taking HRT alters a woman's risk of problems in the womb lining (endometrium) (see Chapter 5). The first test is usually a scan.

**Ultrasound scans.** A scan is usually done from within your vagina, but can also be done through your tummy wall. It will look at the womb and the ovaries. It looks not only at the endometrium, but also will check for fibroids or cysts on your ovaries.

**Biopsy.** A biopsy or small sample of tissue may need to be taken from the lining of the womb. A biopsy is usually done without an anaesthetic by passing a fine tube through the neck of the womb and obtaining the tissue with gentle suction. The procedure is similar to having a smear. You may have some period-like pain during and after the procedure. In some cases, however, the biopsy is obtained under general anaesthetic usually as a day case and has been called a D&C or dilatation and curettage.

**Hysteroscopy.** A hysteroscopy is direct viewing of the inside of the womb. It involves passing a fine telescope inside the womb through the neck of the womb and can either be done without or with a general anaesthetic.

| Test | Might be used . . . |
|------|---------------------|
| FSH (follicle stimulating hormone) level in blood | if your doctor is unsure whether your menopause has started, or if your ovaries are not working properly, usually done if you are under 45 |
| Oestradiol in blood | to see how well you are absorbing or responding to oestradiol, eg, from an implant, patch or gel |
| Thyroid function in blood | because thyroid problems are easily confused with menopausal symptoms |
| Catecholamines or 5 hydroxyindolacetic acid in urine | to exclude rare causes of hot flushes (phaeochromocytoma and carcinoid syndrome) |
| Methylhistamine in urine Red cell tryptase in blood | to exclude a very rare cause of hot flushes (mastocytosis) |

Table 4.1. The tests which your doctor might use at the menopause.

## Tests for osteoporosis

Scans to test the density of bone are not recommended for healthy women. However, they can be useful for women at high risk of osteoporosis or who are already thought to have brittle bones (see chapters 3 and 10).

**Scans using x-rays.** The scans generally use x-rays at two different energies to separate and identify soft-tissue and bone. The process has thus been called dual-energy x-ray absorptiometry (DXA). This can accurately measure the mineral density of the bone. This technique is considered to be the "gold standard" method. In order to reduce the risks of repeated x-rays, bone scans are usually only repeated after about three years, although a second scan may be given one or two years after a new treatment has been started to measure its effects. Single-energy x-ray absorptiometry is commonly used for wrist scans.

**Scans using ultrasound.** Ultrasound systems are also being developed to measure heel bone. The machines used have the advantage of being portable and not using x-rays; however, they need further testing before they are used more widely. Their main role is to help identify women at high risk of osteoporosis, rather than diagnosing the condition or following up women on treatment.

**Blood or urine tests.** In future, it may also be possible to diagnose osteoporosis from a blood or urine test by looking at chemicals associated with bone build-up or break-down. Such a test should be able to detect changes such as response to treatment much more quickly (and safely) than bone scans. These bone markers have been identified in the laboratory but are not yet available for routine use.

## Sources of information

**Journal articles**
Medverd JR, Dubinsky TJ. Cost analysis model: US versus endometrial biopsy in evaluation of peri- and postmenopausal abnormal vaginal bleeding. Radiology 2002; 222: 619-627.

Smith-Bindman R, Kerlikowske K, Feldstein VA, et al. Endovaginal ultrasound to exclude endometrial cancer and other endometrial abnormalities. JAMA 1998; 280: 1510-7.

**Web sites**
Department of Health . Quick reference primary care guide on the prevention and treatment of osteoporosis 1998. Department of Health, PO Box 410, Wetherby LS23 7LN. www.open.gov.uk/doh/osteop.htm

# CHAPTER 5
# HORMONE REPLACEMENT THERAPY (HRT)

Over 50 forms of hormone replacement therapy (HRT) are currently available offering different doses, combinations and routes of taking the hormones. The various types or formulations are listed in national formularies such the British National Formulary. Some formularies are available on the internet.

## What is HRT?

Most problems of the menopause are caused by the sudden fall in levels of the female sex hormone oestrogen. The fundamental idea of HRT is therefore to replace the lost oestrogen. However, giving oestrogen alone can be harmful to the womb lining (endometrium) in women who have not had a hysterectomy. So women who have not had a hysterectomy need a second hormone called a progestogen to counteract the effects of oestrogen on the endometrium. HRT can be delivered orally (tablets), transdermally (through the skin), subcutaneously (a long-lasting implant), intranasally (sniffed) or vaginally.

## Oestrogens

Oestrogens are sometimes classified as "natural" or "synthetic", but these terms can be confusing. In this book, we use the term "natural" oestrogens to refer to compounds that can be found naturally in the body, even when they have been manufactured in a laboratory of a pharmaceutical company. These include oestradiol, oestrone and oestriol, which are usually prepared from extracts of soya beans or yams. Horse or equine urine is another common source of HRT hormones; equine oestrogens include about 50-65% oestrone sulphate (the same as the human form) but the rest are equine oestrogens such as equilin sulphate (which does not occur naturally in humans).

Synthetic oestrogens such as ethinyl oestradiol and mestranol, which are used in contraceptive pills, are less suitable for HRT than natural oestrogens because they have a more powerful effect on the body's metabolism.

Table 5.1 below shows the lowest doses that are generally thought to offer protection from osteoporosis. However, there is increasing evidence that lower doses may be just as effective and may cause fewer side effects. However, young women who have an *induced* (surgical) menopause may require higher doses at first to control menopausal symptoms.

### Progestogens

Progestogens are synthetic steroids which share many properties with the female hormone progesterone produced by the ovary (see chapter 1). They are classified according to their chemical structure. There are two main groups of progestogens: those derived from progesterone (dydrogesterone, medroxyprogesterone acetate) and those derived from testosterone (norethisterone, levonorgestrel).

Most are manufactured from plant sources such as yams.

Currently, progestogens are mainly given in tablet form, though

| Oestrogen | Preparation | Minimum dose (per day except for implants) |
|---|---|---|
| Oestradiol | oral | 1-2 mg |
| Oestradiol | patch | 25-50 µg |
| Oestradiol | gel | 1-5 g depending on preparation |
| Oestradiol | implant | 50 mg (every 6 months) |
| Conjugated equine oestrogens | oral | 0.3-0.6 mg |

Table 5.1. Minimum bone sparing doses of oestrogen.

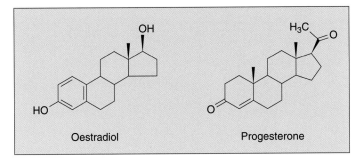

Figure 5.1. Chemical structure of oestradiol and progesterone.

norethisterone and levonorgestrel are available in transdermal patches combined with oestradiol, and levonorgestrel can be delivered directly to the uterus via an intrauterine device (IUD).

The naturally occurring type of progesterone is available as a vaginal gel in the UK. A progesterone pessary for vaginal or rectal use is available but is not currently licensed for HRT. Other progestogens are in development for use in HRT.

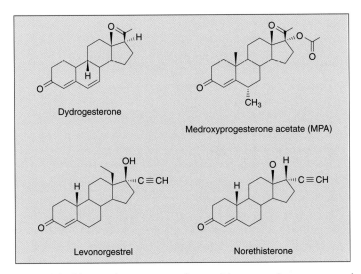

Figure 5.2. Chemical structure of norethisterone, levonorgestrel, dydrogesterone and medroxyprogesterone acetate.

41

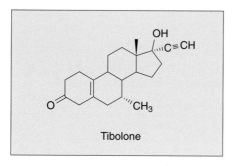

Figure 5.3. Chemical structure of tibolone.

### Tibolone
Tibolone is a synthetic steroid, which has similar effects to both the female hormones oestrogen and progestogen and also the male hormones known as androgens. It is a "no bleed" form of HRT. It can improve psychological and vasomotor symptoms (hot flushes and night sweats) and can increase sex drive (libido). Tibolone can also prevent osteoporosis and the bone sparing dose is 2.5 mg daily. It is a good form of HRT for postmenopausal women who do not want to continue to have periods.

### Androgens (male hormones)
The male hormone testosterone may be used to improve libido. Such treatment is not always successful because sexual problems around the menopause are often caused by several different factors. The current form of treatment is an implant, but testosterone patches and gels are being studied in research trials. They will become available if found to be effective and safe.

### HRT for women who have had a hysterectomy
One in five British women will have had a hysterectomy by the age of 55. The best HRT for women who have had a total hysterectomy, where the whole womb including its neck (cervix) has been removed, is oestrogen alone. Combined HRT (oestrogen plus progestogen) offers no benefits for these women and may increase their risk of breast cancer. However, women who have had a partial (subtotal) hysterectomy, may still have some womb lining (endometrium) present. This will respond to oestrogen alone (see below). To decide whether this is the case, they may be given

| Timing of progestogen | Effect on bleeding |
|---|---|
| 10-14 days every 4 weeks | Monthly bleeds |
| 14 days every 13 weeks | Bleeds every 3 months |
| Continuous | No bleeds |

Table 5.2. The effect of progestogen on bleeding patterns.

sequential HRT first. If they have monthly bleeds, this is an indication that there is some womb lining present. In this case, they should receive combined HRT.

### HRT for women who have <u>not</u> had a hysterectomy

Women who have not had a hysterectomy need both oestrogen and progestogen. The progestogen is added to reduce the risk of benign but excessive growth (endometrial hyperplasia) and cancer of the endometrium, which can be caused by oestrogen alone. Progestogen may be taken cyclically (for a few days every month or every three months) or continuously. How and when the progestogen is taken will have an effect on bleeding patterns, as explained in Table 5.2 above.

Women who have had endometrial ablation (an operation to destroy the endometrium), often performed for heavy periods, should receive progestogen - not all the endometrium will necessarily have been removed and they may be at risk of hyperplasia if they take oestrogen alone.

### HRT around the menopause

Women often notice hot flushes, mood changes and vaginal dryness several months or years before their periods stop (see chapter 1). You do not need to wait for your periods to stop before starting HRT. The best options at this stage are usually monthly cyclic treatments - oestrogen every day with progestogen added for 10-14 days each month. Women with infrequent periods or who get side effects from progestogens may prefer to take the progestogen every three months, and this is called long-cycle HRT. Continuous combined preparations with oestrogen and progestogen every day are not recommended around the menopause because they are likely to cause irregular bleeding.

### HRT after the menopause

One year after the menopause has occurred, many women prefer to switch to continuous combined HRT since this does not cause any bleeding and may reduce the risk of endometrial cancer. This form of HRT is sometimes called "no bleed" HRT. However, it is not always easy for doctors to decide when a woman has reached this stage. Strictly speaking, a woman is considered to be postmenopausal 12 months after her last period, but this can be difficult to determine, especially for women who start to use HRT before their periods stop.

The following may be helpful in deciding when a woman is postmenopausal:

- Age: 80% of women are postmenopausal by the age of 54.
- Earlier lack of periods or raised FSH (follicle stimulating hormone) levels in a blood test (see chapter 1).
- Women whose periods have stopped for six months or who have raised FSH levels in their mid 40s are usually post-menopausal after taking HRT for several years.

Irregular bleeding or spotting can occur during the first 4-6 months of continuous combined HRT and is not a cause for alarm. However, you should consult your doctor if you get heavy (rather than light) bleeding, if it lasts for more than six months, or if bleeding starts suddenly after some time without bleeding. Irregular bleeding may sometimes be improved by increasing the amount of progestogen.

### HRT delivery systems

Any medicine taken by mouth (orally) will go into the stomach and intestines, be absorbed and pass into the liver. This process causes chemical changes to the medicine before it reaches the blood stream. If a medicine is delivered directly into the blood stream (parenterally), these changes are avoided. The route of delivery can therefore influence the effects of medicines and also their side effects. Parenteral delivery systems include skin patches and gels, nasal spray, vaginal rings and implants. Both oral and parenteral systems raise hormone levels throughout the body.

### Oral versus parenteral systems

When HRT is taken orally as tablets, the main type of oestrogen in the blood stream is oestrone. When HRT is taken parenterally the main hormone is oestradiol.

Other differences between oral and parenteral HRT are complex and subtle, and their effects are controversial. Laboratory tests suggest that the route of delivery might affect blood clotting and lipid levels (eg, cholesterol), but the actual effect on women taking different types of HRT is unclear.

Doctors currently debate the advantages of oral and parenteral HRT. There is no clear evidence that one route is better than the other. Many doctors recommend tablets as the first choice for most women unless there is a special reason to prefer another form. However, some will recommend parenteral preparations.

### Parenteral delivery systems

These can used to deliver the oestrogen and in some cases the progestogen. If only the oestrogen is given with a particular system such as a patch, a progestogen will have to be given as well in women who have not had a hysterectomy. The purpose is to protect the lining of the womb. It can be given in various forms such as tablets or an intrauterine coil.

### Transdermal systems: patches and gels

Oestradiol and progestogens can pass into the blood stream through the skin. They can therefore be delivered via transdermal patches or gel.

There are two types of HRT patch. Reservoir patches contain their hormones in an alcohol-based solution and stick to the skin by an adhesive ring at the edge of the patch. Matrix patches contain hormone distributed throughout an adhesive layer, which covers the whole of the patch. Allergic skin reactions are less common with matrix than reservoir patches. Patches are changed either twice or once a week.

Oestradiol is the only form of oestrogen which is available in transdermal form. In the UK, patches, which deliver the progestogens norethisterone or levonorgestrel combined with oestradiol, are available in both monthly sequential and "no bleed" formulations.

### Nasal spray
Oestradiol can be given by a nasal spray and is quickly absorbed into the blood stream (within 10-30 minutes). A daily intranasal dose of 300 μg oestradiol seems to be as good as taking 2 mg/day tablets for treating menopausal symptoms.

### Vaginal ring
Because oestradiol is so well absorbed, some vaginal rings can give blood levels similar to tablets or patches.

### Implants
Small pellets of oestradiol can be placed just under the skin. The insertion is carried out under local anaesthetic. These implants release oestradiol over many months. Implants have the advantage that you do not have to remember to take your medication. However, some women find that their menopausal symptoms return even though the implant is still releasing oestradiol. Levels of oestradiol in the blood may be checked before new pellets are inserted, especially in women coming back more frequently for treatment.

### Intrauterine devices
Devices placed in the uterus (IUDs, sometimes called coils) may be used before the menopause as contraceptives. One type of IUD releases the progestogen levonorgestrel. As well as being a contraceptive, it can therefore be used to deliver progestogen for HRT. The contraceptive effects may be useful in the perimenopause, when women are often still fertile despite having menopausal symptoms. Another advantage is that this method of delivering progestogen is the only one that may not cause bleeding in perimenopausal women. Around 90% of women who have not stopped their periods when it is inserted will be bleed free by 12 months.

## Treating local symptoms without raising hormone levels throughout the body
Some women do not wish to use, or cannot take, systemic HRT (any form which raises hormone levels throughout the body) but they still appreciate relief of symptoms such as dry vagina and

urinary problems. In this case, oestrogens can be given locally to the vagina in the form of a low dose cream, pessary, tablet or ring. These preparations raise local hormone levels but do not affect the whole body. Low doses of natural (rather than synthetic) oestrogens (eg, oestriol or oestradiol) are best for this form of treatment. Progestogen is not needed, since these local doses of oestrogen do not affect the endometrium. Synthetic oestrogens should be avoided because they can enter the blood stream from the vagina. Long-term treatment is usually needed, as symptoms often return when treatment is stopped. Local oestrogen can be used together with systemic therapy if symptoms persist.

## Sources of information

**Journal articles**
Ansbacher R. The pharmacokinetics and efficacy of different estrogens are not equivalent. Am J Obstet Gynecol 2001; 184: 255-263.

Monthly Index of Medical Specialities. Haymarket Medical Ltd, London UK (appears monthly).

Notelovitz M, Lenihan JP, McDermott L, et al. Initial 17β-estradiol dose for treating vasomotor symptoms. Am J Obstet Gynecol 2000; 95: 726-731.

Rymer J, Morris EP. Extracts from clinical evidence: menopausal symptoms. BMJ 2000; 321: 1516-1519.

Varila E, Wahlstrom T, Rauramo I. A 5-year follow-up study on the use of a levonorgestrel intrauterine system in women receiving hormone replacement therapy. Fertil Steril 2001; 76: 969-973.

**Web sites**
British National Formulary. http://bnf.vhn.net/home.

## CHAPTER 6
# BENEFITS AND RISKS OF HORMONE REPLACEMENT THERAPY

Nearly all the important long-term complications of the menopause are caused by lack of oestrogen. Replacing oestrogen through hormone replacement therapy (HRT) is therefore the only treatment that addresses the cause of the problem rather than simply reducing the symptoms.

Many women get great benefits from HRT, both for their menopausal symptoms and for their long-term health. However, it can also cause problems, and it may carry longer term risks.

### Benefits of oestrogen therapy
The many possible benefits of oestrogen replacement are listed in Table 6.1 on the opposite page. Because some of these are controversial we have also set out in the text which follows the evidence about them, where it is available.

### Short-term benefits
**Vasomotor symptoms**
Relieving hot flushes, particularly those occurring at night, will help to improve a woman's sleep pattern and hence reduce irritability, insomnia and tiredness. Hot flushes and night sweats usually improve dramatically within four weeks of starting HRT. The maximum effect of any type of HRT is usually seen by three months, so this is a good point to review the treatment. Treatment should be continued for at least one year, otherwise symptoms often recur.

**Short-term benefits**
- Reduces vasomotor symptoms (eg, hot flushes)
- Improves psychological symptoms (eg, mood swings)

**Long-term benefits**
- Maintains bone mass and reduces the risk of fracture
- May affect risk of cardiovascular disease (heart attack and stroke) but this is highly debated
- May reduce the risk or delay the onset of Alzheimer's disease
- Reduces urogenital problems (eg, dry vagina, bladder problems)
- Reduces the risk of bowel cancer
- May improve wound healing
- May improve balance and reduce falls
- May reduce tooth loss
- May reduce the risk of developing eye diseases of old age such as cataracts and macular degeneration
- May protect against arthritis

Table 6.1. The benefits of taking HRT.

### Psychological benefits

Many women experience an improvement in their psychological well-being after starting HRT. The cause of this is controversial.

Oestrogen may reduce depression directly and restore flagging vigour and confidence. HRT can often dispel a wide range of psychological problems such as disturbed sleep, loss of interest in sex, tiredness, oversensitivity, tearfulness and feelings of guilt and aggression. HRT may therefore be the first choice of treatment (rather than antidepressants, tranquillisers or sleeping tablets) for menopausal women who experience these symptoms.

However, for some women, the side effects of using HRT can outweigh the advantages. These can include painful breasts, nausea and bloating. These effects can increase rather than help psychological distress.

If you suffer side effects from using HRT, you should discuss these with your doctor or health professional. A different dose or preparation may suit you better.

There may be other explanations why women feel better when they take HRT.

• It is simply reassuring to discover that your symptoms can be explained. Even women who receive a dummy treatment (placebo) in research studies often report that they feel better.

• Many psychological problems are linked to other symptoms. If HRT reduces a woman's hot flushes at night, and helps her to sleep better, she will feel better and have more energy in the daytime. There is evidence that women who do not have vasomotor symptoms report less psychological improvement with HRT.

• Even women who do not have a mood disorder, such as depression, report an increased sense of well-being and confidence with HRT, especially if they have had a surgical menopause.

• Oestrogen may have a direct antidepressant effect. In one study of severely depressed psychiatric patients oestrogen improved depressive symptoms regardless of menopausal status.

• Oestrogen can relieve problems that will affect a woman's sex life such as vaginal dryness (which can make intercourse uncomfortable). Some women also experience improved libido. However, it is not a "cure all" for all relationship problems.

## Long-term benefits
### Osteoporosis (brittle bones)
Oestrogen taken in adequate doses (listed in Chapter 5) will stop bone loss. During the first 18-24 months of taking HRT the bone mass should actually increase. After this it usually levels off. Some progestogens, such as norethisterone, may enhance the effects of oestrogen. Tibolone also protects bones.

Bone protection only lasts for as long as the HRT is taken. As soon as it is stopped, the bone loss starts again. It used to be assumed that a woman's risk of breaking her hip would be reduced by the amount of time she took HRT. However, recent studies suggest that 5-10 years of HRT soon after the menopause does not significantly reduce the risk of hip fracture 30 years later. Most hip fractures occur in women aged over 80. The most recent research suggests that lifelong use of HRT or other treatment (see chapter 8) is required to prevent hip fractures.

Most studies have measured the effects of HRT on bone density rather than on the number of fractures. However, two studies have shown a clear effect on spine (vertebral) fractures. Women who already have one vertebral fracture are at high risk of suffering another. They may therefore get particular benefit from HRT. A large randomised controlled trial (The Women's Health Initiative) showed that HRT reduced the risk of hip fracture. Combining results from several studies shows that HRT also reduces other types of fractures (eg, at the wrist).

The standard doses of different oestrogens believed to protect bone are shown in Chapter 5. However, it is now clear that lower doses offer similar protection. It is also now becoming apparent that some women have no bone response despite taking HRT as recommended, but the reasons for this are uncertain. Women who smoke or are very thin seem to be most likely not to respond.

## Cardiovascular disease

Heart attacks and strokes are a major cause of death in women. It is therefore important to know the effects of HRT on these two diseases. Until recently most doctors believed, based on the available evidence, that HRT definitely reduced the risk of heart attacks and possibly strokes. There also appeared to be no difference between the use of oestrogen alone and oestrogen combined with progestogen. This has now been questioned following recent studies showing that HRT did not prevent heart attacks or strokes in women with or without cardiovascular disease. A small increase in heart attacks and strokes was reported in some studies. This area is highly debated and is likely to remain so for many years. This section will try and clarify the various issues involved in this controversial subject.

### Coronary heart disease (CHD)
### Primary and secondary prevention studies of heart disease

Two types of studies can be undertaken: preventing heart disease in healthy women (primary prevention) or preventing further disease in women whose coronary arteries are already blocked (secondary prevention).

### What types of studies have been undertaken?

The effects of HRT on the heart and blood vessels have been looked at in various ways. Studies have measured its effects on lipid levels (eg, cholesterol), blood clotting, blood vessel linings (endothelial function), or sensitivity to insulin in humans and in animals. While levels of these factors are related to heart attacks, they are only markers of disease.

Similarly studies looking at the effect of HRT on the development of blocked and hardened arteries (atherosclerosis) only produces a limited amount of information since not all women with narrowed arteries have heart attacks.

Thus, population or epidemiological studies have been designed to find out if there are any differences in the rates of heart disease between HRT users and non-users. One problem with this type of study is that women who use HRT may be more health-conscious, with better lifestyles in terms of diet and exercise, than non-users. In order to overcome this problem, randomised trials have been set up in which half the women, allocated by chance, get HRT, and the other half get a dummy treatment (placebo); the results are then compared between the two groups.

Overall, until now, primary and secondary prevention randomised trials have not shown that HRT reduces the risk of heart attacks. However, it has been suggested that certain groups of women, such as those with high blood lipid levels, may benefit. Only one type of HRT has been studied extensively so far and it is not known if others might have different effects. This is certainly possible, since different HRT preparations may have different effects on the risk factors for CHD.

**What does "risk" mean?**
Studies often report their results as *relative* risks; however, this can be hard to understand.

For example, a relative risk of 2 could describe something that increases the risk of a disease from one in a million to two in a million, or something that increases the risk of a disease from four people in ten to eight people in ten. In order to understand what a relative risk means, you therefore have to know how common a disease is (which is known as the *absolute* risk).

Relative risks only describe the size of the increase in risk without telling you how large the absolute risk is. Thus, a small increase in relative risk for a common disease (large absolute risk) can have a big effect on the number of people affected, yet a larger increase in relative risk for a very rare event (small absolute risk) will have only a tiny impact on the number affected.

The increases in the relative risk of CHD (29%) found in the Women's Health Initiative primary prevention study in women taking oestrogen and progestogen were widely quoted in the media. But the absolute risk increase, although significant, is fairly small. The true increased incidence of heart attacks for women taking HRT is 0.09%. Thus, out of 10,000 women taking HRT each year there would be seven extra heart attacks compared with a group of 10,000 women who were not taking it.

**What are the limitations of the studies?**
One problem in trying to measure the effects of HRT is that women who use HRT may be more health-conscious and lead healthier lives than non-users. Randomised trials try and get over this, but women taking part in such studies have chosen to do so and may not be typical of the whole population. In addition, in randomised controlled trials there may still be differences between the groups studied - for example, in the number of smokers, or the proportion who take other medications that can reduce CHD.

Another concern is that the age of women in the studies and their other health conditions make it difficult to make the findings relevant to most HRT users. For example, in some trials most participants were in their 60s, but most women who take HRT are in their early 50s. Furthermore, the doses of oestrogen used by women in their 50s to relieve hot flushes is higher than that needed, or tolerated, by older women. Studies of older women with heart disease have used inappropriately high doses of oestrogen, which could in part account for the observed lack of benefit.

**What do we know about the different types of HRT?**
The continued survival of the human race over several million years implies that female sex hormones themselves are not dangerous to health. However, it must be remembered that findings of trials only apply to the particular type of HRT studied. Most of the randomised trials have examined only conjugated equine oestrogens combined with one progestogen, medroxy-progesterone acetate, given by mouth. We therefore know very

little about other oestrogens and progestogens in different dose combinations (especially lower doses) or giving HRT parenterally (see chapter 5). The findings may not be the same for other types of HRT. It is quite likely that HRT using different oestrogens and progestogens, and various routes of administration, would have similar effects on the breast, bowel and bones. But the metabolic or biochemical effects of various HRTs are clearly different, and this is likely to impact on their cardiovascular effects. That's why it is important that studies are carried out using different types of HRT.

The effects of HRT on CHD are therefore unclear.

The following guidelines for doctors about HRT and cardio-vascular disease are based on those from the American Heart Association:

**Secondary prevention** (ie, women who already have cardiovascular disease (CVD))
● HRT should not be started solely in order to prevent CVD
● The decision to continue or stop HRT in women with CVD should be based on other known benefits and risks and on the patient's preference
● If a woman taking HRT develops CVD or becomes immobile (eg, confined to bed), you should consider stopping HRT, or giving treatment to prevent deep blood clots, while she is in hospital. The decision about whether to restart HRT when she leaves hospital should be based on non-CVD benefits and risks, and the patient's preference.

**Primary prevention** (ie, in women without cardiovascular disease (CVD))
● There is not enough evidence to support the use of HRT solely to prevent CVD. Decisions about using HRT should therefore be based on other known risks and benefits.

**Stroke**
Evidence about the effects of HRT on the risk of stroke is unclear. There have been few randomised trials and they have the same limitations as the CHD studies. Population studies are hard to interpret because they do not separate different kinds of stroke

(caused by blood clots or bleeding). Some studies also lump together current HRT users with women who once used HRT but have now stopped. The Women's Health Initiative primary prevention randomised study of women taking combined oestrogen and progestogen found that for 10,000 women taking HRT each year, compared to those not taking HRT there would be an additional eight strokes. A randomised trial of women who had already had one stroke (caused by a blood clot) found that HRT did not reduce the risk of having another stroke or of dying.

### Alzheimer's disease

Alzheimer's disease (AD) is becoming a major worldwide problem as people live longer. One in ten retired people will develop dementia (or a serious loss of mental function) and this rises to one in five people aged over 80. Alzheimer's disease is more common in women than in men, and women also live longer.

Lack of oestrogen may play a role in AD. Some of the building blocks of oestrogen come from fatty tissue and these are particularly important after the menopause when the ovaries stop producing oestrogen. AD is more common in thin women who lack this source of oestrogen. It is also more common in women who have had a heart attack or a hip fracture, suggesting that low oestrogen could be a common risk factor for these conditions.

The effects of oestrogen on the brain are unclear. It seems to increase the production of chemical messengers (neuro-transmitters), reduce the production of some lipids and increase blood flow. Several population studies have suggested that HRT may delay or prevent the onset of AD. The effects seem to be related to the oestrogen dose and the length of use. Women who have taken oestrogen tend to get AD later in life than those who have not.

Laboratory studies suggest that oestrogen improves nerve cell function and reduces the build-up in the brain of the protein amyloid, which is linked to AD. It also seems to protect the brain from the effects of these amyloid deposits. However, in women who already have AD, HRT does not seem to slow its progress or to improve thinking or overall functioning. Thus, it seems that, while HRT may prevent women from developing dementia, it does not alter the disease when it is already established.

55

### Age-related changes in memory and thinking
Before-and-after studies suggest that taking HRT may improve thinking and memory in healthy postmenopausal women, especially in those who have had a surgical menopause. However, HRT probably does not prevent normal, age-related memory loss.

## Changes in urinary and reproductive organs
The changes that take place in the urinary and reproductive tissues after the menopause are called urogenital atrophy. They can cause symptoms such as vaginal dryness and urinary problems (see Chapter 3). It may take up to a year for these symptoms to respond to oestrogen therapy. Fortunately, vaginal problems often respond to low dose directly applied local oestrogen therapy (see Chapter 5). This has advantages over combined oestrogen and progestogen for women who have not had a hysterectomy since it does not cause any bleeding.

Urinary symptoms usually require systemic therapy with tablets or patches. Problems of urgency, frequency and needing to pass water at night (nocturia) are often relieved by HRT. However, stress incontinence (leaking urine when you exercise, laugh, cough or sneeze) cannot be cured by HRT alone, but may respond to a combination of oestrogen and other medicines.

Oestrogen may prevent recurrent urinary tract infections but the correct dose and length of treatment for this are not yet clear.

### Bowel (colorectal) cancer
There is now good evidence from randomised trials that HRT reduces women's risk of getting bowel cancer, but the reason is unclear. For 10,000 women taking HRT each year compared to those not taking it, there would be six fewer bowel cancers.

## Other benefits
HRT may also improve wound healing and postural balance and reduce tooth loss. Women who use HRT are less likely to suffer from cataracts and macular degeneration which are leading causes of blindness in older people. A recent study suggested that long-term HRT use might protect against arthritis. This is interesting since many women complain of aches and pains in their joints at the menopause, which usually respond to HRT.

## Risks of oestrogen therapy

As we have seen, HRT offers many benefits. Yet, as with any medicine, it also carries risks. In deciding whether to use HRT you need to weigh up the benefits and the risks and think about how they apply to you individually.

The three major risks linked with HRT are:

● Breast cancer
● Endometrial cancer, which affects the lining of the womb
● Deep venous blood clots (venous thromboembolic disease)

The risk of ovarian cancer with HRT has become controversial recently and will also be discussed.

## Breast cancer

Breast cancer is a common disease with a lifetime risk in the UK of 1 in 10. Each year, about two women in every 1000 aged between 50 and 70 will develop breast cancer. Understandably, women are concerned about any factors which may increase their risk. However, the proportion of women who survive breast cancer has increased considerably over the last 20 years. This is mainly due to the more widespread use of therapies such as tamoxifen and chemotherapy.

The NHS mammographic breast screening programme is also leading to the earlier diagnosis of smaller cancers. The most recent figures show that of the 39,000 women diagnosed with breast cancer annually in the UK 12,000 die of their disease; this means that over two-thirds are cured.

### HRT and breast cancer risk

Many of the studies that have looked at the relationship between breast cancer and HRT are hard to interpret, as they are population studies which lack control groups for comparison and may be biased. However, there is now some evidence from randomised trials, which compare women taking HRT with others using placebo. Such studies provide more reliable evidence about the risks and benefits of HRT.

As with cardiovascular disease, it may be helpful to think more about the absolute risk of breast cancer than the differences between HRT users and non-users (relative risk). An explanation of these risks is given in Table 6.1 on the next page.

We do know that the earlier a woman has her menopause, the lower her risk of developing breast cancer. This suggests that breast cancer risk depends on how long a woman produces oestrogen. Overall, studies show that HRT has a similar effect to a late menopause. Without using HRT, a woman's risk of getting breast cancer increases by 2.8% for every year that her menopause is later than the average. Similarly, HRT increases the risk of breast cancer by 2.3% for every year it is used. However, this increased risk is not seen among women who start HRT at a younger age for a premature menopause. Available evidence reveals that short-term use of HRT (ie, for less than five years) does not increase risk.

### Types of HRT and breast cancer risk
At one time, doctors thought that adding progestogen to oestrogen would cancel out the increased risk of breast cancer. However, combined results from many studies have shown that this is not the case. In fact, several studies have shown that women using combined HRT have a somewhat higher risk of breast cancer than those using oestrogen alone. There is therefore no reason to give progestogen to women who have had a hysterectomy.

It is possible that different progestogens or the way in which they are taken (cyclic or continuous) may have different effects - but the evidence about this is still confusing. Even if adding a progestogen to the oestrogen raises the risk of breast cancer slightly, this has to

| Length of HRT use | Additional breast cancers per 1000 women using HRT | | |
|---|---|---|---|
| | 2 years | 5 years | 10 years |
| Oestrogen alone | 0.7 | 2 | 5 |
| Combined HRT | 2 | 8 | 22 |

Table 6.1. Estimated numbers of extra breast cancers with oestrogen-alone or combined HRT use for 2, 5 and 10 years.

be weighed against the definite benefits of protection against cancer of the endometrium (see pages 60 and 61).

To get these figures in perspective, it is helpful to compare the risk attributed to HRT with other known risk factors for breast cancer:

| Risk factor | Increase in breast cancer risk |
|---|---|
| Periods starting before 11 | 1.50 x increase |
| Menopause after 55 | 2.00 x increase |
| Postmenopausal obesity | 1.60 x increase |
| Not having a child before 30 | 1.90 x increase |
| Alcohol (more than 2-3 units per day) | 1.50 x increase |
| HRT for more than 5 years | 1.35 x increase |

The increased risk of breast cancer with HRT declines after it is stopped. Five years after stopping HRT a woman's risk of breast cancer is no greater than for women who have not taken it.

If women are taking HRT at the time that their breast cancer is diagnosed, their survival (life expectancy) does not appear to be reduced. It is not known whether this is because cancers are diagnosed at an earlier stage in HRT users or because it has a favourable effect on the type of cancer that develops.

**HRT and women at high risk of breast cancer**
**Women with a family history.** There is little evidence whether HRT further increases the risk of breast cancer in women with a family history of the disease. Information from a relatively small number of studies suggests that there is no added risk, although more studies are needed.

If you are concerned about a family history of breast cancer you should discuss this with your doctor. If necessary you can be referred to the local breast unit for advice and perhaps genetic counselling.

**Women with a personal history of a benign breast disorder.**
Benign breast disorders cover a wide range of conditions, most of which do not increase the risk of cancer. Available studies suggest that HRT does not appear to increase breast cancer risk in women with benign breast disorders. However it may cause breast cysts and breast discomfort.

**HRT after breast cancer**
The use of HRT by women who have had breast cancer is controversial. The most difficult aspect is the management of oestrogen deficiency symptoms as there are so few alternatives to HRT. Symptoms, such as hot flushes and vaginal dryness, are the most common side effect of breast cancer treatment. Breast cancer patients are five times more likely to experience symptoms than healthy postmenopausal women and the symptoms last for longer and may be more severe.

The most commonly used alternatives to HRT consist of either prescription medicines or complementary therapies (see chapters 8 and 9). Unfortunately, very few of these have been evaluated in placebo-controlled trials; the studies are often too short (weeks rather than months) and do not account for possible interaction with breast cancer treatments given at the same time. An added issue for women who have been treated for breast cancer is the fact that some alternatives act like oestrogen. In the absence of any clear evidence about their safety, uncertainty prevails.

In the absence of effective alternatives, many patients have been prescribed HRT to reduce their symptoms. Several small studies have been published and to date none has shown that the use of HRT after breast cancer is associated with a worse survival. Three large randomised trials are now under way to test the use of HRT further; one is being done in the UK. Breast cancer patients suffering from oestrogen deficiency symptoms should take guidance from their local oncology or menopause clinic.

**Endometrial cancer**
Endometrial cancer is much rarer than breast cancer with fewer than 1 in 1000 women in the UK over the age of 50 developing it. The link between unopposed oestrogen replacement therapy and endometrial cancer was established over 20 years ago. Women who have not had a hysterectomy are therefore usually prescribed a combined preparation of oestrogen and progestogen. This has been shown to reduce the risk of both benign and cancerous growth of the endometrium. Women with diabetes or who are obese have an increased risk of endometrial cancer, and this increase is larger than that seen with HRT.

The main symptoms of endometrial cancer are heavy or

unexpected bleeding. You should therefore tell your doctor if you experience these while using any form of HRT. You should also tell your doctor if you have any unexpected bleeding after the menopause, even if you are not taking HRT.

### Endometrial cancer and oestrogen alone
Systemic oestrogen taken on its own significantly increases the risk of endometrial cancer in women who have not had a hysterectomy. This increased risk remains for at least five years after stopping oestrogen. Low-dose vaginal use of oestrogen does not carry this increased risk.

Use of unopposed oestradiol or conjugated oestrogens increases the risk of endometrial cancer about six times. The increase appears to be less (about three times) with low-potency oestrogens such as oestriol taken orally. The increase is reduced by cyclic use of progestogens, and virtually disappears when continuous progestogen is added to the oestrogen.

### Endometrial cancer and oestrogen with added progestogen
There is clear evidence that adding progestogen to oestrogen therapy reduces the effect of oestrogen on the endometrium. However, the evidence is not so clear about how much progestogen needs to be added. At least 10 days per month are recommended for monthly cyclical dosing, but it does not reduce the risk of endometrial cancer down to baseline. It is also not clear whether a three-monthly progestogen cycle offers significantly less protection than monthly use.

No increased risk of endometrial cancer has been found with continuous combined or "no bleed" regimens, so these are probably best for postmenopausal women.

### HRT after endometrial cancer
Whether a woman who has had endometrial cancer should use HRT depends on the extent and type of the tumour. Recent evidence suggests that HRT does not increase the rate of recurrence or death among endometrial cancer survivors. You should take advice from a specialist menopause clinic. In some cases progestogen alone may be helpful, and this treatment is safe for women who have had endometrial cancer.

61

## Deep blood clots (venous thromboembolic disease)

Venous thromboembolism (or VTE) occurs when veins become blocked by blood clots. This is quite different from coronary artery thrombosis, when an artery in the heart becomes blocked. Although we have known for some time that the contraceptive pill increases the risk of VTE, a link with HRT has been shown only relatively recently. The baseline risk of VTE in menopausal women is about 1 in 10,000 per year. Using HRT increases this risk between two and four times. So, for every 10,000 women who use HRT each year, we would expect two extra cases of VTE. For every 100 women who develop VTE, one or two will die.

It remains unclear exactly why HRT affects the risk of VTE. HRT affects some of the substances involved with blood clotting, and transdermal HRT seems to have less effect than tablets. However, the overall risk of VTE is low and in general the benefits of HRT are likely to outweigh the small increase.

### HRT and women at high risk of VTE

**Previous VTE or family history.** Women at most risk of VTE are those who have had VTE in the past. You should tell your doctor if you have ever had VTE, and especially if you were given anti-coagulant treatment for this, such as warfarin. The relevance of a positive family history (ie, having close relatives who have had VTE) is unclear, and it is probably less important than your personal history. Nevertheless you must tell your doctor about this.

Once you have had a VTE, you are at increased risk of having another one even if a blood clotting test is normal after antico-agulant treatment has been stopped. Moreover, women who have previously suffered a VTE have an increased risk of developing another when taking HRT.

**A tendency to blood clotting.** If you have a condition which encourages blood clotting - such as Factor V Leiden, a mutation of the prothrombin gene, antithrombin deficiency or an acquired antiphospholipid syndrome - you may be advised to avoid HRT unless you take an anticoagulant. Women with fewer risk factors, such as a positive family history or a minor problem with blood clotting, need to consider the risk of VTE but can usually use transdermal HRT safely.

**Surgery, HRT and VTE**
If you have to go into hospital for surgery, the doctor will assess your risk of VTE but there is often no need to stop using HRT.

## Ovarian cancer
A possible link between HRT and cancer of the ovary is currently attracting attention, but no clear conclusions can be drawn from the current evidence. There is a possible slightly increased risk from very long-term use (more than 10 years) of oestrogen alone, but there is no clear evidence about the effects of combined preparations or shorter use.

## Possible side effects of HRT
Both the oestrogen and the progestogen in HRT can cause unwanted effects. Some of these are short-lived and usually disappear after a couple of months, but others may be more troublesome. You should discuss any side effects with your doctor or nurse.

You are more likely to experience side effects if you start HRT some time after your ovaries have stopped producing oestrogen. The most common side effects are:

- Tender or painful breasts
- Fluid retention causing bloating and weight gain
- Nausea (feeling sick)
- Headaches
- Leg cramps
- Stomach upsets (indigestion)
- Mood swings/low mood
- Acne
- Backache
- Lower abdominal (belly) ache

Many of these side effects will wear off after you have been using HRT for three months. If side effects continue to be troublesome there are various solutions. For example, gamolenic acid can help reduce breast tenderness.

Leg cramps can improve with lifestyle changes, such as avoiding standing up for long periods of time.

Nausea or upset stomach may be reduced by changing the time you take your HRT in relation to mealtimes. You might also try switching from oral HRT (tablets) to another route such as patches.

If problems persist, your doctor might suggest trying a different type of oestrogen or progestogen, or a different route of delivery (eg, patch, gel, nasal spray, vaginal ring, implant). A change in dose might also help; however, you still need enough oestrogen to prevent menopausal symptoms and/or bone loss, and enough progestogen to prevent unwanted growth of the womb lining unless you have had a hysterectomy.

Progestogen given as continuous combined therapy (daily with oestrogen) often causes fewer side effects than when given cyclically, but this method of HRT is only suitable for women once they are postmenopausal (one year after their last natural period, as explained in chapter 5).

**Weight gain**
Many women are reluctant to start or continue with HRT because they think they will put on weight. In the first few months some women do notice some fluid retention, which can cause them to feel bloated, but several carefully designed studies comparing HRT to dummy treatment have repeatedly shown no evidence that HRT causes weight gain overall. However, it is true that most women, whether or not they take HRT, do put on some weight after the menopause.

**Bleeding**
If you take sequential or cyclical HRT, you will normally get a predictable pattern of light bleeding towards the end or soon after the end of the progestogen phase. Tell your doctor if you have bleeding that is heavy, longer than usual, irregular or painful. Changing the type or dose of progestogen may help, but your doctor will also need to check that there is no other cause. A few women (about 5%) using sequential HRT have no bleeding and it is not a reason to worry. No bleeding is usually because the womb lining is very thin, but in the perimenopause you should also make sure that you are not pregnant (see the section on contraception in Chapter 10).

Breakthrough bleeding (bleeding at unexpected times) is

common with both continuous combined and long cycle (3-monthly progestogen) HRT in the first 3-6 months of treatment. Tell your doctor if you get breakthrough bleeding after this time.

## How long should you take HRT?

This is an individual decision, but will depend on your medical history.

● If you take HRT mainly to prevent menopausal symptoms it is usually a good idea to stop after five years to see if the symptoms return. If not, you can stop taking HRT. This length of use will not significantly increase your risk of developing breast cancer.

● If you are concerned about preventing or treating brittle bones (osteoporosis) you should consider taking HRT for the rest of your life. A recent population study suggests that taking HRT for 5-10 years soon after the menopause does little to reduce your risk of breaking your hip 30 years later. If you are concerned about the disadvantages or risks of long-term HRT you could consider other agents such as bisphosphonates to treat osteoporosis ( see chapter 8). If you are at risk of osteoporosis (see chapter 3), having your bone mineral density measured can help you decide whether you should have long-term treatment of some sort.

● If you had an early (premature) menopause (see chapter 1) you should take HRT until the average age of the natural menopause - in other words, until you are 51. After this, the issues discussed above will apply and you should discuss this with a health profes-sional.

## Sources of information

**Journal articles**
Cholerton B, Gleason CE, Baker LD, Asthana S. Estrogen and Alzheimer's disease: the story so far. Drugs Aging 2002; 19: 405-427.

Grady D, Herrington D, Bittner V, et al. Cardiovascular disease outcomes during 6.8 years of hormone therapy: Heart and Estrogen/progestin Replacement Study follow-up (HERS II). JAMA 2002; 288: 49-57.

Herrington DM, Howard TD, Hawkins GA, et al. Estrogen-receptor polymorphisms and effects of estrogen replacement on high-density lipoprotein cholesterol in women with coronary disease. N Engl J Med 2002; 346: 967-974.

Hextall A. Oestrogens and lower urinary tract function. Maturitas 2000; 36: 83-92.

Lacey JV Jr, Mink PJ, Lubin JH, et al. Menopausal hormone replacement therapy and risk of ovarian cancer. JAMA 2002; 288: 334-341.

Nelson HD, Humphrey LL, Nygren P, Teutsch SM, Allan JD. Postmenopausal hormone replacement therapy: scientific review. JAMA 2002; 288: 872-881.

Rosendaal FR, Vessey M, Rumley A, et al. Hormonal replacement therapy, prothrombotic mutations and the risk of venous thrombosis. Br J Haematol 2002; 116: 851-854.

Santen RJ, Pinkerton J, McCartney C, Petroni GR. Risk of breast cancer with progestins in combination with estrogen as hormone replacement therapy. J Clin Endocrinol Metab 2001; 86: 16-23.

Soares CN, Almeida OP, Joffe H, Cohen LS. Efficacy of estradiol for the treatment of depressive disorders in perimenopausal women: a double-blind, randomized, placebo-controlled trial. Arch Gen Psychiatry 2001; 58: 529-534.

Torgerson DJ, Bell-Syer SE. Hormone replacement therapy and prevention of nonvertebral fractures: a meta-analysis of randomized trials. JAMA 2001; 285: 2891-2897.

La Vecchia C, Brinton LA, McTiernan A. Cancer risk in menopausal women. Best Pract Res Clin Obstet Gynaecol 2002; 16: 293-307.

Writing Group for the Women's Health Initiative Investigators. Risks and benefits of estrogen plus progestin in healthy postmenopausal women: principal results from the Women's Health Initiative randomized controlled trial. JAMA 2002; 288: 321-333.

**Web sites**
A number of reviews are available from the Cochrane Library web site (http://www.cochrane.org), for example:
MacLennan A, Lester S, Moore V. Oral oestrogen replacement therapy versus placebo for hot flushes. Cochrane Database Syst Rev 2001; (1): CD002978.
Hogervorst E, Yaffe K, Richards M, Huppert F. Hormone replacement therapy to maintain cognitive function in women with dementia. Cochrane Database Syst Rev 2002; (3): CD003799.

National Library of Medicine. Medline Plus Health Information on Menopause
http://www.nlm.nih.gov/medlineplus/menopause.html

Royal College of Physicians. Osteoporosis: clinical guidelines for prevention and treatment. Update on pharmacological interventions and an algorithm for management. London, Royal College of Physicians 2000.
http://www.rcplondon.ac.uk/pubs/wp_osteo_update.htm

## CHAPTER 7
# THE MENOPAUSE AND OTHER MEDICAL CONDITIONS

Female hormones affect many body systems, so the menopause can affect other conditions such as diabetes and migraine. Talk to your doctor if you have concerns about this. In some cases, it may be helpful to get advice from a specialist clinic. This chapter outlines the main conditions that are likely to be affected by the menopause and might affect your decision about taking HRT. A summary of the effects of HRT appears in Table 7.2 at the end of this chapter.

## Gynaecological (women's) problems
### Fibroids
Fibroids are non-cancerous growths in the muscle wall of the womb (myometrium). They are affected by oestrogen levels and often shrink after the menopause. However, they can increase with oestrogen, so HRT may cause heavy or painful bleeds. The effects of different types of HRT on fibroid growth are unclear. Your doctor may use ultrasound or a pelvic examination to assess the size of the fibroids occasionally.

### Endometriosis
Endometriosis is a condition in which the tissue lining of the womb (endometrium) grows in the wrong places, sometimes forming cysts.

Endometriosis may be treated by removing the excess tissue, which sometimes may involve removing one or both ovaries (oophorectomy). It may also be treated by drugs to reduce oestrogen production called GnRH analogues (eg, buserelin, goserelin). In theory, HRT can re-activate the disease, even after surgery. The risks, however, appear to be small. Some gynaecologists avoid giving oestrogen alone, especially for the first six months after oophorectomy. Instead of oestrogen they may recommend a progestogen on its own, continuous combined oestrogen and progestogen therapy or tibolone to control vasomotor symptoms. There is no clear evidence about which of these is best.

Women who have had endometriosis may be at particular risk of the long-term effects of low oestrogen levels caused either by the GnRH analogues or oophorectomy.

### Cancer and abnormal growth (dysplasia) of the cervix
These are not affected by oestrogen levels, so it is safe to use HRT.

## Cardiovascular disease
### High blood pressure (hypertension)
There is no evidence that HRT raises blood pressure or does any harm to women with hypertension. Severe hypertension is a very rare side effect of conjugated equine oestrogens, but blood pressure returns to normal when treatment is stopped.

### Diseases affecting the heart valves
HRT can safely be used by women with valvular heart disease. Those taking anticoagulants sometimes have problems with irregular or heavy bleeding. This can usually be resolved by adjusting the progestogen dose.

### Raised blood lipids (hyperlipidemia) and cholesterol
High levels of lipids (fats) in the blood are a risk factor for heart attacks and strokes. The most important lipids in this respect are LDL (low density lipoprotein), triglyceride and lipoprotein(a). In contrast, HDL (high density lipoprotein) protects against heart disease (see chapter 3). Different types of HRT have different effects on blood lipids. If you have raised lipid levels, your doctor should tailor your HRT to your individual needs. HRT can safely be taken with statins, which are drugs which lower blood lipid levels. Table 7.1 on the next page summarises the effect different types of HRT have on lipid levels.

| | HDL (good) | LDL (bad) | Triglyceride | Lipoprotein(a) |
|---|---|---|---|---|
| Ideal HRT | ↑↑ | ↓↓ | ↓↓ | ↓↓ |
| Oral oestrogen | ↑ | ↓↓ | ↑ | ↓↓ |
| Transdermal oestrogen | - | ↓ | ↓ | ↓ |
| Oral progesterone derived progestogen | ↑ | ↓ | ↑ | ↓ |
| Oral testosterone derived progestogen | - | ↓ | ↓ | ↓ |
| Tibolone | ↓ | ↓ | ↓↓ | ↓ |
| Raloxifene | - | ↓ | - | ↓ |

↑ small increase    ↓ small decrease
↑↑ big increase    ↓↓ large decrease

Table 7.1. Effects of hormones on lipid levels.

### Diabetes and thyroid disease (endocrine diseases)
### Diabetes mellitus

Many specialists now believe that HRT is important for postmenopausal women with diabetes. A woman's risk of developing diabetes increases sharply after the menopause and the number of postmenopausal women who have diabetes is rising. Women with diabetes are at increased risk of coronary heart disease (CHD). Women of South Asian origin are at higher risk of both diabetes and CHD than Europeans, so preventing heart disease is doubly important for them.

There are two types of diabetes. Type 1 usually starts in childhood and needs to be treated with insulin. Type 2 occurs later in life and usually does not need insulin. Women with type 1 diabetes have lower bone density in middle age than women without diabetes or those who have type 2 diabetes. Preventing osteoporosis is therefore particularly important for these women.

Until recently, many doctors had concerns about prescribing HRT for women with diabetes. Some information about HRT advised caution in cases of diabetes. However, opinions have changed, and the North American Menopause Society (NAMS) has issued a helpful statement which recommends using transdermal oestrogen preparations, or oral oestrogens in low dose. The choice of progestogen is less clear but micronised progesterone or dydrogesterone seem to have the least unwanted effects on insulin sensitivity and HDL cholesterol levels.

### Thyroid disease

An overactive thyroid gland (hyperthyroidism) is linked with an increased risk of osteoporosis and hip fractures. Women with hyperthyroidism should therefore be screened for osteoporosis. Women receiving thyroxine treatment for an underactive thyroid (hypothyroidism) may also be at risk of osteoporosis. Thyroxine can be taken with HRT, but the dose may need to be increased since oestrogen can affect thyroxine absorption.

## Neurological conditions

### Migraine

More women than men suffer from migraine, and the headaches usually start during their teens and twenties. It is unusual for migraines to start after the age of 50.

Many women with migraine get headaches around their monthly period. Migraine often improves after a natural menopause, but may get worse after a surgical menopause (bilateral oophorectomy) unless HRT is given. There is no good evidence that HRT makes migraine worse.

Because migraine can be triggered by changes in oestrogen levels, skin patches or vaginal rings are probably better than tablets since they produce more stable hormone levels. Too much oestrogen can trigger migraine aura (flickering lights that many people see before the headache starts) but this usually resolves if the dose is reduced. Unlike the contraceptive pill, there is no evidence that women with migraine who take HRT are at increased risk of stroke. Cyclic monthly progestogen may trigger migraine headaches in some women. Changing the type of progestogen, changing to continuous combined therapy, or giving the progestogen in a patch or via an intrauterine device may solve the problem (see chapter 5).

### Epilepsy

There is not much information about the effects of the menopause and HRT on epilepsy. Some anti-epileptic medicines may affect the way in which HRT is broken down in the liver, but there are no studies to show whether transdermal HRT is better than oral or whether women taking these medicines should take a higher dose of HRT. Some anti-epileptic drugs such as phenytoin and carbamazepine can cause decreased bone mass and increase the risk of osteoporotic fractures.

### Parkinson's disease

Population studies suggest that taking oestrogen after the menopause may reduce the risk of Parkinson's disease. The effects of HRT on women with Parkinson's disease are limited, but it appears to be safe, and may even help the symptoms.

## Gastrointestinal (gut) problems

### Gall bladder disease

About one in 12 people in the UK aged over 40 has gall stones, and this figure rises to more than one in five of those aged over 60. However, there is not much information on the effects of HRT on gall stone formation. Some population studies and a recent randomised trial of oral HRT in elderly women suggest that those taking it are more likely to have gall bladder disease. Many doctors recommend parenteral forms of HRT for women with gall bladder problems, but there is little evidence to support this.

### Liver disease

Most doctors recommend a non-oral route of HRT so that oestrogen enters the blood stream directly and does not first go via the liver. However, evidence to support this theory is limited. Some types of liver disease such as primary biliary cirrhosis are linked with osteoporosis. Specialist advice may be helpful.

### Crohn's disease

Women with Crohn's disease may be at increased risk of osteoporosis either from the disease itself or because of long-term treatment with corticosteroids. Transdermal HRT is usually preferred to ensure it is properly absorbed.

## Coeliac disease

Bone density is reduced in coeliac disease and nearly half of all women on gluten-free diets will develop osteoporosis. This is probably caused by an inability to absorb calcium and possibly also vitamin D. HRT is therefore important to reduce the risk of bone fractures. Transdermal routes may be better than oral.

## Autoimmune diseases

### Rheumatoid arthritis

Rheumatoid arthritis is caused when the body forms antibodies to tissues in the joints; this causes them to become inflamed, swell up and be painful. Rheumatoid arthritis is different from the more common form, osteoarthritis, which is largely caused by physical wear and tear on the joints as you get older. The main symptoms of rheumatoid arthritis are inflamed, painful joints. Women are affected about 2.5 times more often than men.

Women with rheumatoid arthritis are at increased risk of osteoporosis. This may be because of steroid treatment, lack of exercise as a result of stiff and painful joints, and the fact that the disease itself can cause bone loss. There is no evidence that using HRT affects the risk of developing rheumatoid arthritis. In women who already have the disease, there is no evidence that HRT makes it worse. Many women are advised to take HRT as their doctors feel that osteoporosis will simply compound their problems.

### Systemic lupus erythematosus (SLE)

SLE is a rare disease of the immune system affecting many body systems including the heart and kidneys. SLE usually gets worse during pregnancy, suggesting that hormone levels affect it.

Long-term use of steroids means that women with SLE are at high risk of osteoporosis. Studies have shown that one in eight SLE patients will have fractures, and their fracture rate is nearly five times higher than normal. Women with SLE should therefore benefit from anything that reduces osteoporosis. However, many doctors believe that SLE is affected by oestrogen, and that HRT will increase the rate of flares. There are few studies in this area to support or disprove these ideas, so HRT should be considered with caution. SLE may also affect blood clotting, and HRT is usually not suitable for women at risk of venous thrombosis (see chapter 6).

## Other conditions
### Asthma
Women taking HRT seem to be at slightly greater risk of developing asthma and symptoms such as wheezing. However, for most women who already have asthma HRT does not seem to make it worse.

### Otosclerosis (conductive deafness)
This is an inherited condition which causes progressive deafness. The condition seems to get worse during pregnancy, and, occasionally, when sufferers take the contraceptive pill. However, there is no evidence that HRT makes it worse. Since the disease is naturally progressive, hearing will gradually get worse in long-term HRT users, just as it does in non-users as they get older.

### Skin cancer (malignant melanoma)
This is a controversial area. Most doctors accept that there is no link between using HRT and a woman's risk of getting malignant melanoma. Studies about the effect of HRT on the outlook for women who do get skin cancer are contradictory. This type of cancer does contain oestrogen receptors, but it is unlikely that the oestrogen in HRT increases its growth.

Age spots (dark patches on the skin) are most common on people in their 70s. They are usually found on the cheek or neck, and are linked to exposure to sunlight and ultraviolet (UV) radiation. Some types of age spot (called lentigo maligna) can turn into skin cancer. Pre-cancerous cells contain receptors for both oestrogen and progesterone, which suggests that levels of these hormones might affect the transformation from benign to cancerous growth.

### After a transplant
Bone mass often falls following an organ or bone marrow transplant because of treatments given to prevent rejection of the transplant. Up to 80% of transplant patients will have osteoporosis (brittle bones) and up to 65% will have a fracture. Bone loss is largely due to the use of steroids (glucocorticoid therapy) after the transplant but may also be linked to immunosuppressive treatment (eg, cyclosporin A or tacrolimus). There is not much information about the use of HRT in women who have received a transplant,

| Condition | Risk of osteoporosis for women with this condition | The effect of HRT |
|---|---|---|
| Asthma | Increased in long-term oral steroid users | May increase risk slightly, slight or no effect on existing condition |
| Cervical cancer and dysplasia | | Safe to use |
| Crohn's/coeliac disease | Increased | Transdermal route is best |
| Diabetes | Increased | Safe to use |
| Endometriosis | | Small increased risk of disease reactivation |
| Epilepsy | Increased by phenytoin and carbamazepine | Safe to use but dose may be affected by antiepileptic medication |
| Fibroids | | Can cause enlargement |
| Gall bladder problems | | May increase risk of disease slightly |
| High blood pressure | | Safe to use |
| Hyperlipidemia (high lipids) | | Safe to use, type depends on lipid profile |
| Kidney failure | Increased | Should be considered |
| Liver disease | Can be increased | Transdermal route preferred, seek specialist advice |
| Migraine | | Safe to use, transdermal is best |
| Otosclerosis | | Probably safe |
| Parkinson's disease | | Safe to use, may reduce risk of getting disease |
| Post-transplant | Increased | Should be considered |
| Rheumatoid arthritis | Increased | No increase in flares |
| Skin cancer (malignant melanoma) | | Not linked with increased risk |
| Systemic lupus | Increased | No increase in flares |
| Thyroid disease | Increased | Safe to use |
| Valvular heart disease | | Safe to use |

Table 7.2. HRT for women with different medical conditions.

but it should probably be considered, along with other measures to reduce osteoporosis.

### Kidney (renal) failure

Patients with kidney failure (sometimes called end-stage renal disease or ESRD) are at increased risk for an early menopause, osteoporosis, mental and heart disease. However, few postmenopausal women with kidney failure receive HRT. More information is needed to understand the benefits and risks of HRT for these women.

## Sources of information

**Journal articles**

Abbasi F, Krumholz A, Kittner SJ, Langenberg P. Effects of menopause on seizures in women with epilepsy. Epilepsia 1999; 40: 205-210.

Arafah BM. Increased need for thyroxine in women with hypo-thyroidism during estrogen therapy. N Engl J Med 2001; 344: 1743-1749.

Bousser MG, Conard J, Kittner S, et al. Recommendations on the risk of ischaemic stroke associated with use of combined oral contraceptives and hormone replacement therapy in women with migraine. The International Headache Society Task Force on Combined Oral Contraceptives & Hormone Replacement Therapy. Cephalalgia 2000; 20:155-156.

Colacurci N, De Franciscis P, Cobellis L, et al. Effect of hormone replacement therapy on postmenopausal uterine myoma. Maturitas 2000; 35: 167-173.

Delmas PD. Osteoporosis in patients with organ transplants: a neglected problem. Lancet 2001; 357: 325-26.

Godsland IF. Effects of postmenopausal hormone replacement therapy on lipid, lipoprotein, and apolipoprotein (a) concentrations: analysis of studies published from 1974-2000. Fertil Steril 2001; 75: 898-915.

Green PS, Simpkins JW. Neuroprotective effects of estrogens: potential mechanisms of action. Int J Dev Neurosci 2000; 18: 347-58.

Hallengren B, Elmstahl B, Berglund J, et al. No increase in fracture incidence in patients treated for thyrotoxicosis in Malmo during 1970-74. A 20-year population-based follow-up. J Intern Med 1999; 246: 139-144.

Lange P, Parner J, Prescott E, Ulrik CS, Vestbo J. Exogenous female sex steroid hormones and risk of asthma and asthma-like symptoms: a cross sectional study of the general population. Thorax 2001; 56: 613-616.

Matorras R, Elorriaga MA, Pijoan JI, et al. Recurrence of endometriosis in women with bilateral adnexectomy (with or without total hysterectomy) who received hormone replacement therapy. Fertil Steril 2002; 77: 303-308.

Mosca L, Collins P, Herrington DM, et al. Hormone replacement therapy and cardiovascular disease: a statement for healthcare professionals from the American Heart Association. Circulation 2001; 104: 499-503.

North American Menopause Society. Effects of menopause and estrogen replacement therapy or hormone replacement therapy in women with diabetes mellitus: consensus opinion of The North American Menopause Society. Menopause 2000; 7: 87-95.

Persson I, Yuen J, Bergkvist L, Schairer C. Cancer incidence and mortality in women receiving estrogen and estrogen-progestin replacement therapy- -long-term follow-up of a Swedish cohort. Int J Cancer 1996; 67: 327-332.

Scott EM, Gaywood I, Scott BB. Guidelines for osteoporosis in coeliac disease and inflammatory bowel disease. British Society of Gastroenterology. Gut 2000; 46 Suppl 1: 11-18.

Scuteri A, Bos AJ, Brant LJ, Talbot L, Lakatta EG, Fleg JL. Hormone replacement therapy and longitudinal changes in blood pressure in postmenopausal women. Ann Intern Med 2001; 135: 229-238.

Smith MA, Fine JA, Barnhill RL, Berwick M. Hormonal and reproductive influences and risk of melanoma in women. Int J Epidemiol 1998; 27: 751-757.

Thompson W. Otosclerosis and hormone replacement therapy: fact or fiction? J Br Meno Soc 1999; 5: 54.

# CHAPTER 8
# ALTERNATIVES TO OESTROGEN THERAPY

Women who do not want or who are unable to take oestrogen can consider other options to treat their symptoms and prevent the long-term effects of the menopause.

## Preventing and treating osteoporosis (brittle bones)
## Drug treatments
### Bisphosphonates

Bone consists of a honeycomb-like framework onto which minerals such as calcium are deposited. Bones lose density when these minerals are no longer deposited, or by an active process of breakdown called resorption. Bisphosphonates are taken up at sites where the bone minerals are deposited and form stable compounds, which resist breakdown.

Bisphosphonates are not easily absorbed from the gut, especially if it contains food, and so should always be taken on an empty stomach. However, they may occasionally irritate the gut and cause symptoms of indigestion. These symptoms stop quickly if you stop taking the bisphosphonate.

Several different bisphosphonates are available. Etidronate, alendronate and risedronate are the ones most often used to prevent and treat osteoporosis; their chemical structure is shown in Figure 8.1 on the following page. They are also effective for osteoporosis associated with corticosteroid use (see chapter 3).

Women who can take oestrogen may benefit from taking both a bisphosphonate and oestrogen. This combination has a greater effect on bone density than either agent alone. Bisphosphonates given by injection are in development.

**Etidronate** has been widely studied in postmenopausal osteoporosis. There is solid evidence that it can prevent fractures of the spine, but less strong indications that it also prevents hip fractures. Usually, 400 mg of etidronate is taken for 14 out of every 90 days, and calcium (1250 mg) is taken for the other 76 days. It may seem strange, but taking etidronate continuously rather than in 14-day sessions actually increases bone loss. There is no limit to the length of time this treatment can be taken.

**Alendronate** has a stronger effect than etidronate and there is solid evidence that it can prevent both spine and hip fractures. Unlike etidronate it may be taken either every day or once weekly. Doses of 10 or 20 mg daily have been shown to strengthen bones in the spine and hips. The greatest increase is seen in the first year, and it reaches a plateau after two or three years. Bone mass is preserved for at least one year after treatment is stopped. Clinical studies have shown that women taking alendronate had half as many fractures as those who were not taking it. The dose needed to prevent osteoporosis is 5 mg daily. The dose for treating established disease is either 10mg daily or 70 mg once a week. Once weekly dosing may be more convenient and side effects are less common.

**Risedronat**e, like alendronate, is more potent than etidronate. There is solid evidence that it reduces spine and hip fractures. In

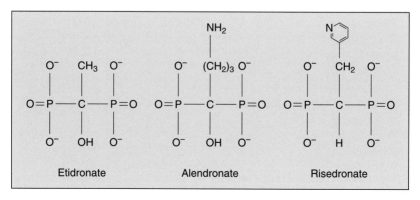

Figure 8.1. The chemical structure of bisphosphonates.

women with established osteoporosis 5 mg of risedronate taken daily for three years reduces the risk of new fractures by between a third and a half. It can also be given once weekly. The dose is 35 mg.

**Calcium and vitamin D**
Whatever treatment is used to prevent or treat osteoporosis, it is important that women get enough calcium and vitamin D, either from food or as a supplement. British women, especially the elderly, often lack vitamin D. Most of our vitamin D comes from the action of sunlight on the skin. Good dietary sources include oily fish, fortified cereals and soft spreads such as margarines. Lack of sunlight is an issue for women who tend to be covered up when they go outdoors, or never go out at all, such as those in residential care. Because of Britain's northerly position, the skin only produces vitamin D in the summer, and our national diet lacks sufficient vitamin D to make up for this. In other countries, even those with more sunshine such as the USA, dairy products are fortified with vitamin D.

High doses of calcium and vitamin D have been shown to decrease the rate of bone loss in elderly postmenopausal women. Calcium supplements of 1000 mg or more taken daily may decrease bone loss in women with osteoporosis. There is strong evidence that high amounts of calcium decrease the risk of spine

| Food | Amount | Calcium content (mg) |
| --- | --- | --- |
| Full-fat milk | 250 ml | 295 |
| Semi-skimmed milk | 250 ml | 300 |
| Skimmed milk | 250 ml | 305 |
| Low-fat yoghurt | 100 g | 150 |
| Cheddar cheese | 50 g | 360 |
| Boiled spinach | 100 g | 159 |
| Brazil nuts | 100 g | 170 |
| Salmon (tinned) | 100 g | 93 |
| Tofu | 100 g | 480 |

Table 8.1. The calcium content of foods.

fracture, but the evidence on hip fracture is less strong. Additionally, vitamin D and calcium supplements decrease the risk of hip and other fractures in the frail elderly, and is therefore recommended for them. The benefits of taking vitamin D without calcium are less clear.

The current UK recommended daily dose of calcium is 700 mg. However, most studies show that women need around 1500 mg (ie, more than twice this amount) to keep their bones healthy after the menopause if they are not taking HRT. A lower dose of 1000 mg is enough for women who are using HRT. Most studies have been on elderly women, and there is no evidence that calcium alone (without HRT) can reverse bone loss around the menopause.

Women who do not want or who are unable to take calcium supplements should be careful to include calcium-rich foods in their diet. Table 8.1 on the previous page shows the calcium content of some foods.

### Calcitriol
This is a natural substance formed in the body by the breakdown of vitamin D. It helps calcium to be absorbed from food and also has direct effects on bone cells. The results of studies on fractures are unclear and thus this preparation is not often used in the UK. Also people taking calcitriol need their calcium levels checked.

### Selective oestrogen receptor modulators (SERMs)
The hormone oestrogen acts by binding to cellular receptors. Different receptors occur on different types of cell. Some substances therefore affect the oestrogen receptors on some cells but not others. Some chemicals even have opposite effects in different tissues and organs. These are called selective oestrogen receptor modulators, or SERMs (the acronyn refers to the American spelling which is estrogen). One of the first SERMs was tamoxifen, which is widely used to treat breast cancer. Tamoxifen acts against the effects of oestrogen in the breast but strengthens the effects of oestrogen on bones and lipids. It is not licensed to treat or prevent osteoporosis, and is usually only prescribed for this by specialist units.

Raloxifene was the first SERM to be licensed to prevent spine fractures caused by osteoporosis. Its chemical structure is

Figure 8.2. The chemical structure of raloxifene.

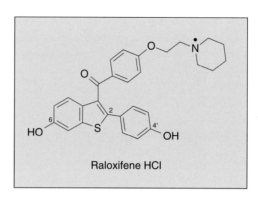

Raloxifene HCl

illustrated in Figure 8.2. Raloxifene has been available in the UK since 1998. It is only suitable for postmenopausal women.

Studies have shown that women who took raloxifene (60 mg per day) for two years had significantly greater bone mineral density in their spines and hips than women who had taken a dummy treatment (placebo). In women who already have osteoporosis raloxifene can reduce spine fractures by between a third and a half, depending on the dose, but it does not seem to reduce the risk of fractures in other bones such as the hip.

Raloxifene can cause short-term side effects such as hot flushes and calf cramps. It does not treat the symptoms of the menopause and is therefore not suitable for women with hot flushes. Like HRT, it increases the risk of deep blood clots (VTE) (see chapter 6). However, it protects the bone without affecting the womb lining (endometrium) or the breast. It therefore does not cause any bleeding or breast tenderness. It also reduces the risk of breast cancer in women with osteoporosis.

Raloxifene is probably most useful for women aged 60-75 who are at high risk of spine fractures but who cannot, or prefer not to, take HRT. There is strong evidence that it can reduce the risk of spine fractures.

Raloxifene also appears to reduce harmful cholesterol (see chapter 7), but we do not yet know whether this can reduce the risk of heart disease. There is little published information on whether raloxifene can reduce symptoms such as vaginal dryness or discomfort.

**Calcitonin**
Calcitonin controls the balance between bone formation and breakdown. It cannot be taken by mouth, but is available as an injection or nasal spray. Injections are expensive and often cause side effects such as sickness, diarrhoea and hot flushes and may cause allergic reactions. Nasal calcitonin has been shown to reduce fractures of the spine and reduce the pain caused by them. There is also some evidence that it can reduce the risk of hip fractures. It is not available in all countries.

**Parathyroid hormone**
Parathyroid hormone is produced by four small glands found in the neck, near the thyroid. People whose glands are overactive (a condition called hyperparathyroidism) suffer from bone loss, but if parathyroid hormone is taken in short pulses it seems to have the opposite effect.

A study of over 1600 postmenopausal women with osteoporosis showed that the use of parathyroid hormone was associated with a significant decrease in the risk of fractures in the spine and elsewhere - so parathyroid hormone looks like being a major advance in the treatment of osteoporosis. Taken together with HRT, parathyroid hormone is likely to be important for patients with severe osteoporosis.

**Statins (lipid lowering drugs)**
Statins are used to reduce the levels of lipids such as cholesterol in the blood, and so reduce the risk of heart attacks and strokes. However, recent information from animals suggests that statins may also reduce the risk of fractures. This is an intriguing observation, but population studies in humans have produced conflicting results.

**Fluorides**
Fluoride can help to build up bone and is used in toothpaste to strengthen the teeth. Although fluoride can increase bone density in the spine, this does not always seem to be translated into a reduction in the risk of breaking a bone. It has never been shown to prevent hip fractures. Therefore, the use of fluoride for osteoporosis is currently not recommended.

### Strontium ranelate

The benefits of low doses of stable strontium in the treatment of osteoporosis were reported almost 50 years ago. However, it may have been neglected, due to confusion between normal, stable strontium and the radioactive variety. There is some evidence that it may reduce fractures of the spine.

### Non-drug treatments

### Hip protectors

Wearing padding around the hips can lessen the impact of a fall. Wearing a padded plastic hip protector has been shown to reduce the risk of breaking a hip. However, most people find hip protectors rather unattractive and uncomfortable in hot weather, and they are not easy to fit. They are, alas, not particularly attractive.

### Exercise

Weight-bearing exercise such as walking can increase bone mass. People who take exercise regularly have higher bone mass and a lower risk of fracture than those who do not. There is not much evidence that exercise can prevent bone loss around the menopause; however it has other benefits, and can be helpful for women who already have osteoporosis.

The main benefits of exercise are probably increased well-being, muscle strength, better posture and balance and a reduction of aches and pains rather than a direct effect on the bone. Exercise for people with osteoporosis needs to be carefully planned to prevent causing further fractures.

### Preventing and treating falls

Most fractures of brittle bones, apart from those in the spine, are caused by falls. The risk of falling increases with age and is greater in women than in men. HRT with oestrogen appears to improve muscle strength and co-ordination.

Care should be taken if elderly people are taking sedatives or other medicines which may cause drowsiness or confusion, since these can increase the risk of falling.

## Reducing vasomotor symptoms (eg, hot flushes)

● Progestogens such as norethisterone 5 mg/day or megestrol acetate 40 mg/day can help to control hot flushes and night sweats. At this dose norethisterone may also protect the bones a little, but there is no information about whether megestrol acetate does the same. However, both these hormones in the doses detailed above increase the risk of deep blood clots (VTE).

● There is growing evidence that a group of drugs originally developed for people with depression and called selective serotonin-reuptake inhibitors (SSRIs) can reduce hot flushes. SSRIs such as venlafaxine, fluoxetine and paroxetine may therefore be useful for women who cannot take oestrogen - such as those who have had breast cancer.

● The beta-blocker propanolol (widely used to treat high blood pressure) was once recommended for women with hot flushes, but it is now rarely used because studies of its effects have produced conflicting results.

● Clonidine is licensed for treating hot flushes, but it is of limited use and may cause unpleasant side effects.

### Reducing vaginal changes
Simple lubricants can help reduce vaginal dryness and prevent discomfort during sex. However, the effect is short-lived. Longer acting "bioadhesive" moisturisers are now available, and these may also help prevent infections by restoring the protective acidic pH.

## Sources of information

### Journal articles
Bisphosphonates for osteoporosis. Drug Ther Bull 2001; 39: 68-72.

Loprinzi CL, Barton DL, Rhodes D. Management of hot flashes in breast-cancer survivors. Lancet Oncol 2001; 2: 199-204.

Meunier PJ, Slosman DO, Delmas PD, et al. Strontium ranelate: dose-dependent effects in established postmenopausal vertebral osteoporosis - a 2-year randomized placebo controlled trial. J Clin Endocrinol Metab 2002; 87: 2060-2066.

Neer RM, Arnaud CD, Zanchetta JR, et al. Effect of parathyroid hormone (1-34) on fractures and bone mineral density in postmenopausal women with osteoporosis. N Engl J Med 2001; 344: 1434-1441.

Rodriguez-Martinez MA, Garcia-Cohen EC. Role of Ca(2+) and vitamin D in the prevention and treatment of osteoporosis. Pharmacol Ther 2002; 93: 37-49.

Van Staa TP, Wegman S, de Vries F, et al. Use of statins and risk of fractures. JAMA 2001; 285: 1850-1855.

### Web sites
A number of reviews are available from the Cochrane Library web site (http://www.cochrane.org), for example,
Gillespie WJ, Avenell A, Henry DA, O'Connell DL, Robertson J. Vitamin D and vitamin D analogues for preventing fractures associated with involutional and post-menopausal osteoporosis (Cochrane Review). Cochrane Database Syst Rev 2001; 1: CD000227.
Parker MJ, Gillespie LD, Gillespie WJ. Hip protectors for preventing hip fractures in the elderly (Cochrane Review). Cochrane Database Syst Rev 2001; 2: CD001255.

National Cancer Institute. http://press2.nci.nih.gov/sciencebehind

The Royal College of Physicians web site includes the College's guidelines for preventing and treating osteoporosis. These are available at:
http://www.rcplondon.ac.uk/files/osteosummary.pdf
and
http://www.rcplondon.ac.uk/pubs/wp_osteo_update.htm

# CHAPTER 9
# COMPLEMENTARY AND ALTERNATIVE THERAPIES

There is little scientific evidence that complementary and alternative therapies can help menopausal symptoms or provide the same benefits as HRT. Yet many women use them, believing them to be safer and "more natural" than products prescribed by their doctor. Each year, Americans are thought to spend around $27 billion on such remedies, and one British survey found that more than one in ten adults had visited a therapist in the previous year. The choice of treatments is confusing and, unlike conventional medicines, not much is known about their safety or side effects or how they may interact with other therapies.

### Phytoestrogens
Phytoestrogens are plant substances that have effects similar to those of oestrogens. Over 300 plants have been found to contain phytoestrogens. They are found in many foods. Preparations vary from enriched foods such as bread or drinks (soy milk) to more concentrated tablets.

The most important groups are called isoflavones and lignans. The major isoflavones are genistein and daidzein. The major lignans are enterolactone and enterodiol. The chemical structure of phytoestrogens is shown in Figure 9.1.

Isoflavones are found in soybeans, chick peas, red clover and probably other legumes (beans and peas). Oilseeds such as flaxseed are rich in lignans, and they are also found in cereal bran, whole cereals, vegetables, legumes and fruit.

Interest in phytoestrogens has been stimulated by the

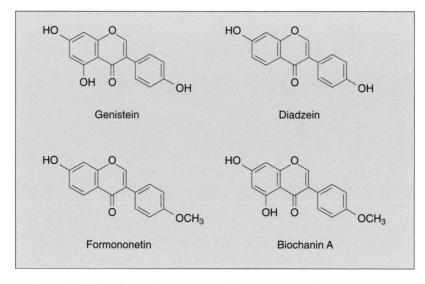

Figure 9.1. The chemical structure of four common phytoestrogens.

observation that women in countries where the diet is rich in isoflavones, such as Japan, seem to have lower rates of menopausal symptoms, heart disease, osteoporosis, and cancers of the breast, large intestine (colon), womb lining (endometrium) and ovary. But it is not straightforward to translate these observations into helpful recommendations for women in other countries since other factors in the Japanese diet might be involved.

When tested in the laboratory, phytoestrogens have been shown to have a variety of properties. They can act like oestrogens, but can also have the opposite effect (anti-oestrogenic). They can kill or reduce the growth of viruses, bacteria and fungi. They may also protect cells against cancer, may lower blood pressure, reduce inflammation, and reduce harmful oxidants.

The most widely studied isoflavone is genistein. In the laboratory it has been shown to have effects on cell division and important cell receptors. It may also stop the formation of new blood vessels around tumours and the process by which normal cells turn into cancerous ones.

There have been few properly conducted studies comparing

phytoestrogens to other treatments or to a dummy treatment (placebo).

Evidence about the effects of extracts of soybean and red clover on menopausal symptoms, blood lipids and blood pressure is confusing. Nevertheless, the US Food and Drug Administration (FDA) allows the makers of certain foods containing soy protein to claim that they reduce the risk of heart disease. There is conflicting evidence about whether phytoestrogens can help maintain bone mass. Phytoestrogens may cause unpleasant and even dangerous side effects. In one study, the synthetic isoflavone ipriflavone caused loss of white blood cells (lymphocytopenia) in a significant number of women.

Further well designed research is needed to discover whether phytoestrogen supplements are effective and safe treatments for women with menopausal symptoms.

## Herbalism

Some herbs (eg, ginseng) have strong oestrogenic properties (ie, they act in the same way as oestrogen), so women who cannot take oestrogen should be very careful when trying herbal treatments. Herbal remedies may also alter the effects of treatments prescribed by your doctor, or cause dangerous side effects. They can interact with blood thinning drugs such as warfarin, antidepressants, drugs used for epilepsy and general anaesthetics. They can either increase or reduce the effects of prescribed treatments.

Another problem with herbal remedies and supplements is that there is little control over their quality and it is often impossible to know exactly what they contain. Some contain high levels of chemicals such as pesticides, arsenic, lead and mercury. Cases of kidney failure, liver failure and even cancer have been linked to herbal treatments.

If you are taking a herbal treatment you must tell your doctor before she/he prescribes a medicine for you.

### Black cohosh

The German authorities have approved the use of black cohosh for some menopausal symptoms. It is known to contain substances that bind to oestrogen receptors, but we do not know if this explains its effects.

### St John's wort

There is good evidence that St John's wort can help some people with mild depression. In a recent study, menopausal women taking St John's wort reported improvements in psychological and psychosomatic symptoms. Most women also noted that their menopausal symptoms reduced or disappeared. However, this study only included women taking St John's wort and there was no comparison group.

Other studies have reported improvements in sexual well-being after treatment with St John's wort extract. St John's wort may increase the effects and side-effects of some anti-depressant drugs (SSRIs), and may affect liver enzymes and therefore alter the effects of HRT.

### Ginseng

Ginseng is a popular therapy for postmenopausal women. However, it has little effect on hot flushes but may improve depression and well-being.

### Oil of evening primrose

Oil of evening primrose contains gamolenic oil and is widely used by women. However, there is at present no evidence that it has any effect on hot flushes, but it may help with breast tenderness.

### Others

Wild yam cream, dong quai, agnus castus (chasteberry), liquorice root, valerian root and ginko biloba are also popular but there is no evidence that they have any effect on menopausal symptoms. Claims have been made that steroids in yams (dioscorea) can be converted in the body to progesterone, but this is biochemically impossible in humans.

### Vitamins and minerals

Vitamins such as E and C and minerals such as selenium are present in various supplements. The evidence that they are of any benefit to postmenopausal women is extremely limited. While one study showed vitamin E to reduce hot flushes, the difference between the active and the dummy treatment (placebo) was only one hot flush per day.

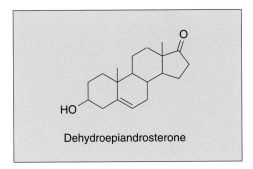

Dehydroepiandrosterone

Figure 9.2. The chemical structure of DHEA.

## DHEA (dehydroepiandrosterone)

DHEA is a naturally occurring steroid produced by cells around the kidneys (called the adrenal glands). Blood levels of DHEA drop dramatically with age. This had led to suggestions that the effects of ageing can be counteracted by DHEA "replacement therapy". DHEA is increasingly being used in the USA, where it is classed as a food supplement, for its supposed anti-ageing effects. Some studies have shown benefits on the skeleton, thought processes (cognition), well-being and the vagina. The short-term effects of taking DHEA are still controversial and possible harmful effects of long-term use are, as yet, unknown.

## Progesterone transdermal creams

Progesterone creams are sold for the treatment of menopausal symptoms and skeletal protection. They have recently been the subject of clinical trials. Women using the cream have reported improvements in vasomotor symptoms (hot flushes, etc) but there was no effect on bone density. Further research is needed to discover whether progesterone creams have any role to play in preventing the long-term effects of the menopause.

Women who have not had a hysterectomy are at increased risk of growths and cancer of the womb lining (endometrium) if they take oestrogen alone (see Chapter 6). Adding a progestogen or progesterone reduces this risk. However, the available evidence suggests that progesterone creams do not provide enough progesterone to offer protection. They should therefore not be used in order to protect the womb lining from the effects of oestrogen.

## Other complementary therapies

Other complementary therapies include acupressure, acupuncture, Alexander technique, Ayurveda, osteopathy, hypnotherapy, reflexology and Reiki. Further research is needed to understand their possible effects. Homeopathy is also popular and some studies suggest it may be of benefit.

## Sources of information

### Journal articles
Kang HJ, Ansbacher R, Hammoud MM. Use of alternative and complementary medicine in menopause. Int J Gynaecol Obstet 2002; 79: 195-207.

Kronenberg F, Fugh-Berman A. Complementary and alternative medicine for menopausal symptoms: a review of randomized, controlled trials. Ann Intern Med 2002; 137:805-13.

Zollman C, Vickers A. ABC of complementary medicine. Complementary medicine in conventional practice. BMJ 1999; 319: 901-904.

### Web sites
National Center for Complementary and Alternative Medicine. Alternative therapies for managing menopausal symptoms. http://nccam.nih.gov/health/alerts/menopause/

The NIH Office of Dietary Supplements (http://dietary-supplements.info.nih.gov)

Office of dietary supplements. IBIDS database. http://ods.od.nih.gov/databases/ibids.html

# CHAPTER 10
# STAYING HEALTHY AROUND AND AFTER THE MENOPAUSE

Even if you go through the menopause with few symptoms, you need to think about your long-term health and it may be helpful to talk to your doctor or practice nurse about this.

Most women take HRT to reduce symptoms such as hot flushes and mood swings, but it can also have long-term benefits such as maintaining healthy bones (see chapter 6). The following groups of women may get special benefit from HRT:
- Those who have an early menopause
- Those with other risk factors for osteoporosis (brittle bones) such as steroid use

You should therefore discuss the possible benefits and risks with your health professional.

If you do decide to use HRT, you need to think about how long you will take it. This is an individual decision as the risks and benefits vary from woman to woman. You should continue with HRT as long as the benefits outweigh the potential disadvantages. There is no fixed time limit on HRT, so you need to discuss this with your doctor to work out what is best for you (see the section in Chapter 6 about how long you should take HRT).

## Looking after yourself
### Diet and lifestyle
A healthy diet and lifestyle are important throughout our lives, but the menopause may be a useful time to review your personal situation.

The huge differences in women's experience of the menopause

around the world may partly be due to variations in diet (including phytoestrogen intake) and lifestyle. A healthy diet and regular exercise are important in protecting against heart disease and fragile bones. Exercise may also reduce vasomotor and psychological symptoms of the menopause such as hot flushes and mood swings. Weight-bearing and muscle-strengthening exercises help to maintain strong bones but the effect is lost as soon as regular exercise stops.

Hot flushes may also be reduced by simple measures such as avoiding heat or drinks containing caffeine or alcohol.

Taking in enough calcium and vitamin D (either in foods or from supplements) is important to maintain healthy bones (see Chapter 8). Other lifestyle changes such as stopping smoking and cutting down on excess alcohol, caffeine, salt and animal proteins may help reduce bone loss and increase calcium absorption. Physical activity, stopping smoking and not being overweight will reduce cancer risk.

Many factors affect the risk of heart attacks and strokes. The most important are probably smoking, blood pressure and lipid levels (cholesterol). Women should identify the factors which may increase their risk, and identify areas of their lives which need alteration.

### Cervical screening
You should continue to have cervical smears (to detect abnormalities or cancer of the womb entrance or cervix) every three years up to the age of about 64. There is no need to have them more frequently or after the age of 64 if you are taking HRT.

### Breast screening (mammography)
A mammogram is a special x-ray of the breast, which can detect breast cancer. At the moment in the UK, women aged 50-64 are automatically invited to have a mammogram every three years. The age band is to be increased to include women up to the age of 70. Older women can request a mammogram every three years. Women at high risk of breast cancer (see Table 10.1 on the next page) should have a mammogram every year from the age of 35 or at five years younger than the youngest relative developed cancer from a minimum age of 30. You should talk to your doctor about

- Four close relatives on the same side of the family have had breast or ovarian cancer at any age (moderate risk)
- Close relative has had both breast and ovarian cancer (moderate risk)
- Three close relatives on the same side of the family have had breast cancer when they were under 70 (moderate risk)
- Mother, sister or daughter had breast cancer when they were under 40 (moderate risk)
- Mother, sister or daughter has had cancer in both breasts (high risk)
- Father or brother with breast cancer (high risk)
- Mother, sister, aunt or grandmother had breast cancer when over 60 (low risk)

Table 10.1. Family risk factors for breast cancer.

any changes in your breasts (lumps, pain or discharge).

There is no indication to have a mammogram before starting HRT and there is no need to have screening mammograms performed more than every three years (the recommended interval between screens in the NHS Breast Screening Programme) for women who are taking HRT.

However, if you develop any new breast symptoms, it is important that you see your doctor whether you are taking HRT or not.

**Unexpected bleeding**
You should tell your doctor about any unexpected change in vaginal bleeding. Your doctor in these cases may arrange for you to have some tests such as a scan or a biopsy to get a small sample of the endometrium (see chapter 4).

## Contraception around the menopause
Just because you have some signs of the menopause, you should not assume that you cannot get pregnant. You should continue to use contraception for two years after your last period if you are

under 50 and for at least one year if you are over 50. Your preferred method of contraceptive may change around the menopause, so information about different methods is presented below.

### Natural family planning
These methods are not reliable around the menopause. At this time your cycle becomes unpredictable, temperature changes are inconsistent, and the nature of the cervical mucous changes. Methods relying on measuring hormone levels at ovulation also become unreliable. To avoid pregnancy you should therefore use another method of contraception

### Coitus interruptus (withdrawal)
This method may be continued if you have used it successfully before. Vaginal dryness, fear of pregnancy and changes in you or your partner's libido and potency may make it more difficult.

### Condoms
You can continue to use these but may find that they make sex uncomfortable. The drier vagina also means that condoms are more likely to split. You should therefore use lubricating or spermicidal gels. Remember that some vaginal preparations such as oestrogen creams and pessaries can weaken condoms and make them more likely to split.

### Diaphragm (cap)
You can continue to use a diaphragm (cap) but changes in the vagina may make it difficult to fit or stay in place. Remember that some vaginal preparations such as oestrogen creams and pessaries can affect the rubber used in diaphragms and make them unreliable.

### Spermicides
Spermicides may make sex more comfortable by increasing lubrication and they are more effective in older women. They can be used alone (eg, foam or pessary) or with a barrier method (eg, diaphragm). Changes to the vagina at the menopause may make you more sensitive to the chemicals in spermicides, so there is more risk of irritation or allergy.

### Intrauterine devices (IUDs /coils)
If you already have an IUD fitted you can continue to rely on it for contraception. It can be left in place until you no longer need contraception.

### Intrauterine systems
IUDs which release the progestogen hormone levonorgestrel offer effective contraception and can also be used to combine with the effects of oestrogen in HRT. They can therefore be used to provide bleed-free HRT for women going through the menopause.

### Combined oral contraceptives (the Pill)
Low dose pills provide reliable contraception as well as the benefits of oestrogen replacement in older women. Women who do not smoke, have normal blood pressure, who are not overweight and do not have a family history of blood clots or breast cancer, can continue using these pills until at least their mid-40s or early 50s. However, they may cause a slightly increased risk of breast cancer and possibly heart attacks and strokes.

### Progestogen only pills (mini-pill)
Progestogen-only pills are suitable for use throughout the perimenopause and there is no upper age limit for their use. In fact, the effectiveness of the mini-pill improves as women get older. There is not much information about the effects of using the mini-pill in combination with HRT.

### Implants (intra-muscular and subdermal progestogens)
If you have an injected or implanted contraceptive, lack of periods can make it hard to tell when the menopause takes place, but they provide reliable contraception and are suitable for use during the menopause. There is not much information about the effects of using them in combination with HRT.

### Sterilisation (male or female)
Sterilisation (vasectomy for the man, or clipping the Fallopian tubes for the woman) is the commonest form of pregnancy prevention in older couples in the UK. It is reliable and has no effect on treatments for the menopause.

## Information your doctor or health professional will need to know

Below is a checklist you can take when you see your doctor to discuss what you want to do about the menopause.

**Periods, symptoms and contraception**
- When was your last period?
- How frequent have your periods been, how heavy and for how long?
- Do you get hot flushes?
- Do you get vaginal dryness?
- Have you any other symptoms?
- What contraception have you and your partner been using?

**Personal or family medical problems**
Tell your doctor if you know about:
- Breast cancer/ovarian cancer in close family members (see Table 10.1)
  - in parents, sisters or brothers or yourself?
  - at what age did they develop it?
- Blood clots in legs (deep vein thrombosis) or lungs (pulmonary embolism) - in parents, brothers or sisters or yourself?
  - when and why: was it after a hip or knee replacement?
  - was the person on the Pill or pregnant?
  - did they have any test to confirm the clot?
  - were they treated with warfarin?
- Risk factors for heart disease and strokes?
  - have you had a heart attack or stroke already ?
  - have your parents, brothers or sisters had a heart attack or stroke and if so at what age?
  - do you smoke and if so how many?
  - do you have high blood pressure or diabetes?
  - do you have a high cholesterol level?
- Risk factors for osteoporosis (see chapter 3 for full list)
  - was your menopause before the age of 45?
  - have you taken corticosteroids for 6 months or more?
  - have you ever been underweight?
  - does it run in the family (especially mother or sister) ?
  - have you had a fracture already; if so how, did it happen and where was it?
- Do you suffer from migraines, not just headaches?
- What medicines are you taking including herbal remedies and vitamin supplements?
- Could you be pregnant?

**What do you want to do?**
- Do you want to take HRT or not?
- If you want HRT, think about which preparation would suit you best.

## Counselling

Many women feel perplexed by the changes in their body and the different treatment options available at the menopause. Getting enough information and having an understanding person to talk to are therefore very important. Your doctor, menopause nurse or pharmacist should tell you about the benefits, risks and possible side effects of any treatments you are being offered. Reassurance and practical advice can often reduce or remove some psychological aspects of the menopause. Other forms of counselling or psychotherapy may be helpful for women whose psychological symptoms are caused by a combination of changes in oestrogen levels and a major life event such as bereavement or separation. Help is available from local self-help groups, bereavement counselling, RELATE (marriage guidance), or assertiveness training.

## Sources of information

**Journal articles**
Peto R, Boreham J, Clarke M, et al. UK and USA breast cancer deaths down 25% in year 2000 at ages 20-69 years. Lancet 2001; 355: 1822.

Rutter CM, Mandelson MT, Laya MB, et al. Changes in breast density associated with initiation, discontinuation, and continuing use of hormone replacement therapy. JAMA 2001; 285: 171-176.

The British Association of Surgical Oncology Guidelines for surgeons in the management of symptomatic breast disease in the UK (1998 revision). Eur J Surgical Oncoclogy 1998; 24: 464-476.

Williams JK. Contraceptive needs of the perimenopausal woman. Obstet Gynecol Clin North Am 2002; 29: 575-888.

**Web sites**
Food standard agency- later life. http://www.food.gov.uk/healthiereating/laterlife/

National Electronic Library For Health. http://www.nelh.nhs.uk/

# WORD LIST

Below are listed some of the frequently used medical terms in this book. Please note that this book uses British spellings. If you get material from the internet you may notice differences in American spellings – if you are searching the internet it is often helpful to try both the British and the American spelling. In general, US doctors use 'e' instead of 'ae' and 'oe' in words such as haemorrhage and oestrogen.

**Anticoagulant:** a medicine that reduces blood clotting
**Artery:** a type of blood vessel
**Atherosclerosis:** narrowing of the arteries due to "furring up" by cholesterol
**Atrophy:** degeneration  or wearing out of a structure

**Biopsy:** a sample of tissue taken for examination
**Bisphosphonates:** a type of medicine used to treat osteoporosis

**Cardiovascular:** relating to the heart and blood vessels
**Cervix:** neck of the womb
**CHD:** coronary heart disease
**Coagulation:** the way and speed at which blood clots
**Colles fracture:** type of fracture of the arm bone near the wrist
**Coronary:** sometimes used as another word for a heart attack, more correctly, the name of the arteries that supply the heart with blood (= coronary arteries)
**Corticosteroid:** prescribed steroids such as hydrocortisone, prednisolone, cortisone and betamethasone

**DVT:** deep vein thrombosis (see venous thromboembolism)
**Dementia:** a serious loss of mental function

**Endometrium:** the lining of the uterus (womb)
**Endothelium:** the inner wall of an artery (plural = endothelia)
**Epithelium:** the surface layer of cells, eg, lining the vagina

**FSH:** follicle stimulating hormone (one of the female hormones produced by the pituitary)

**Haemorrhage:** bleeding
**Haemorrhagic stroke:** stroke caused by bleeding (rather than a blood clot)
**HDL:** high density lipoprotein – a "good" type of cholesterol
**HRT:** hormone replacement therapy
**Hypercholesterolaemia:** raised levels of cholesterol in the blood
**Hyperlipidaemia:** raised levels of lipids (fats like cholesterol) in the blood
**Hypertension:** high blood pressure
**Hysterectomy:** operation to remove the womb
**Hysteroscopy:** procedure to view the inside of the womb

**Ischaemic stroke:** stroke caused by a blood clot or blocked blood vessel

**LDL:** low density lipoprotein – a "bad" type of cholesterol
**LH:** luteinising hormone (one of the female hormones produced by the pituitary)
**Lipid:** fat such as cholesterol
**Lipoprotein(a) (Lpa):** a blood fat
**Lumen:** inside of an organ, eg, a blood vessel

**Menarche:** the time when a girl starts having monthly periods
**Milligram (mg):** one thousandth (0.001) of a gram
**Microgram (µg or mcg):** one millionth (0.000001) of a gram
**Myocardial infarction:** heart attack
**Myometrium:** muscle layer or wall of the womb

**Nocturia:** needing to pass water at night

**Oestrogen:** a female sex hormone produced by the ovary (spelled estrogen in the USA)

**Oocytes:** egg cells
**Oophorectomy:** operation to remove the ovaries
**Oral:** taken by mouth (eg, a tablet)
**Osteoporosis:** a condition in which the bones become very light, fragile, and at risk of breaking
**Ovary:** female reproductive organ

**Parathyroid:** small glands in the neck which produce a hormone which affects calcium metabolism
**Parenteral:** to describe a medicine delivered directly into the blood stream, eg, by a transdermal patch rather than orally
**Placebo:** a dummy treatment (eg, sugar pill) given as part of a clinical study to provide a comparison for the active treatment and to make sure any effects are not simply caused by patients (or doctors) thinking they are getting (or giving) a new form of treatment
**Prolapse:** condition in which the structures supporting organs weaken, causing them to move down in the body (eg, the womb sinks into the vagina)
**Progesterone:** a female sex hormone produced by the ovary
**Progestogen:** synthetic hormone with similar effects to progesterone

**Statins:** a group of drugs that lower cholesterol levels

**Thromboembolism:** blockage of a blood vessel caused by a blood clot
**Thrombus:** a blood clot
**Thyroid:** gland in the neck that produces hormones
**Transdermal:** taken through the skin (eg, an HRT patch)
**Triglyceride:** a blood fat

**Urethra:** the tube that carries urine out of the bladder
**Uterus:** womb

**Vasomotor:** describes symptoms such as hot flushes and night sweats
**Venous thromboembolism:** blockage of a deep vein caused by a blood clot

# INDEX

# About the authors

**Dr Margaret Rees** is a graduate of the University of London and holds a doctorate of philosophy from the University of Oxford. She is a medical gynaecologist and a Reader in Reproductive Medicine in the Nuffield Department of Obstetrics and Gynaecology, University of Oxford. She works in the Menopause Clinic in Oxford, one of the first founded in the UK. Her research focuses on why women have problems with bleeding and on testing new HRT treatments. She is the Editor-in-Chief of the *Journal of the British Menopause Society*. She is married and lives in Oxford.

**Professor David Purdie** is a graduate of Glasgow University Medical School. He is presently Head of Research at Hull University's Centre for Osteoporosis and has a particular interest in the detection and prevention of this brittle bone disease. His research work has included the testing of new HRT treatments and the development of portable bone scanners. He is an advisor to the UK Government on HRT and is a past Chairman of the British Menopause Society. Married to Dr Kate Guthrie, a gynaecologist, Professor Purdie lives in East Yorkshire.

**Dr Sally Hope** is a General Practitioner in Woodstock, Oxfordshire. She has developed a special interest in women's health over the past 20 years. She is an Honorary Lecturer in the Department of Primary Care, University of Oxford. She is a founder member of the Primary Care Group in Gynaecology, and served on the Council of the British Menopause Society for three years. She is a deputy editor of the *Journal of the British Menopause Society*. Dr Hope is married with two teenage girls.